The Courage to Come Back Triumph Over TBI: A Story of Hope

by
Michael Coss

The profits from the sale of this book will be re-directed to The Michael Coss Brain Injury Foundation, which provides Hyperbaric Oxygen treatments that will improve the quality of life of children who need them.

The Courage to Come Back
Triumph Over TBI – A Story of Hope

ISBN 10: 0-9831698-2-9
ISBN 13: 978-0-9831698-2-6

Published by: Expert Author Publishing
http://expertauthorpublishing.com

Canadian Address
1265 Charter Hill Drive
Coquitlam, BC, V3E 1P1
Phone: (604) 941-3041
Fax: (604) 944-7993

US Address
1300 Boblett Street
Unit A-218
Blaine, WA 98230
Phone: (866) 492-6623
Fax: (250) 493-6603

Dedication

This book is dedicated to my children, my son Nathan and my daughter Danielle, as they give me the inspiration and motivation to keep progressing in my rehab. They make me wake up each day on the right side of my bed with a large smile on my face. For them I'm ready, each day, to face the day's challenges that will be thrown my way.

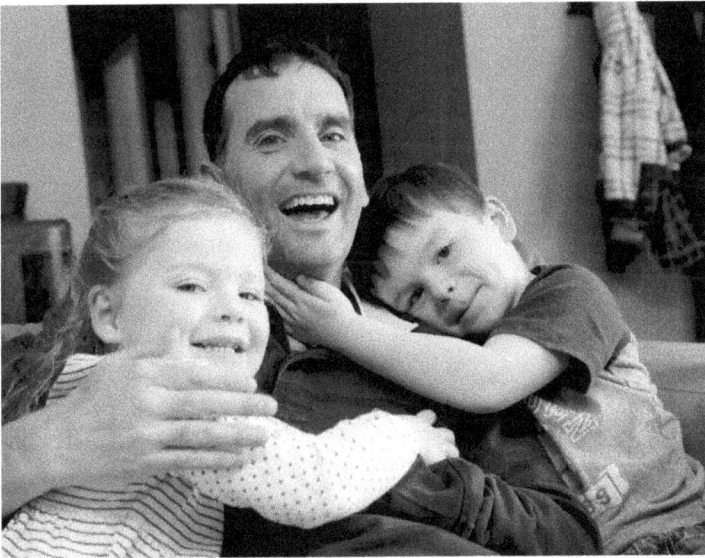

Acknowledgements

I am very fortunate and blessed to have amazing people in my life and I would like to dedicate this book to those people who have made me the person I am today: my parents, my brothers, my wife, my kids, my friends, my co-workers, my teammates on my hockey and softball team, and my customers.

I would like to THANK everyone who touched my life one way: my bosses and former bosses, Don Davis, Ronnie Paterson, Heath Lefroy, David Riggs, Denise Kerr, Maureen Rumley, Kerri Gama, Jay and Jodi Heer, Greg Hutchings, Darren Opsahl, Lynda Perovich, Tim Cowley, Mia Dario, Darcie Prokop, Terry Rollheiser, Terry Filatrault, and Sean Lanigan.

The person, other than my father, who has played one of the largest parts in my life, is my former boss and customer, Ronnie Paterson. He hired me, trained me, and taught me how to win and how to be a leader.

I would like to express my sincere thanks to everyone at The Richmond Hyperbaric Health Center and The Advanced Hyperbaric Recovery Center In Coquitlam.

I would also like to express my sincere thanks to Florence Woo and to her entire team for giving me a second chance at life. I awoke from my close to seven-month deep sleep, my COMA, after just three sessions of HBOT oxygen.

Although I don't have yet full control over my whole body, I have discovered new ways to do things and have adapted quite well considering my traumatic brain injury. New brain pathways are being created. I remain very optimistic that I will one day walk to the park with my children.

A SPECIAL THANKS

I would like to offer a special thanks to my employer, Molson Coors Canada, for hosting my book launch event at its brewery in beautiful Vancouver BC on Wednesday, May 18, 2011. The overwhelming support that my family and I received from Molson Coors Canada is greatly appreciated and does not go unnoticed.

Table of Contents

Forewards

Is recovery from traumatic brain injury possible? This is a question that a great number of individuals whose lives have been altered by traumatic events cope with on daily basis. This is a question that medical professionals and allied health therapists have wrestled with for centuries. I am deeply honored that Michael has asked me to write the foreward for this book. This exceptional story proves that anything is possible through perseverance and character.

A few years ago I received a call at our clinic just outside Montreal, the man I was speaking to identified himself as Bob Coss from Vancouver BC. He continued on to tell me the story of his son Michael who had suffered a severe traumatic brain injury almost year ago as a result of a horrific car accident that had also involved his wife and six month old twins. He went on to explain Michaels ordeal and the primary results they had seen with a therapy called hyperbaric oxygen therapy. The question was should they continue with HBOT and for how long? Is it possible to see more progress if they continue?

My heart went out to Bob and his family as I myself have been on a similar path for the last sixteen years as a parent advocating for their child, leaving no stone unturned as we search for more than the mainstream medical community has to offer and a better quality of life. My story, although very different from the Coss family is built on the determination to help my twin sons who both have cerebral palsy and are legally blind due to a lack of oxygen at the time of their premature birth. Much like Michael we have spent thousands of hours participating in many different therapies over the years. As lives are changed and we are forced to take a new path this is when we find out what we are really made of and how driven and determined we can become.

A good support network can help but it doesn't define recovery. The drive to maximize your quality of life lies within you. In the end it comes down to being the best that you can be. Many in Michael's position would opt to quit and nobody would find fault faced with the monumental task of rehabilitation. Within this book Michael provides a unique perspective of recovery from traumatic brain injury through the eyes of one whose life has changed dramatically. The faith to overcome is that of the person affected. Michael has come a very long way towards healing, yet he is not finished. Along the way he has embraced a number of therapies that many medical professionals dismiss without consideration. Michael's determination has been greatly enhanced by his reluctance to accept what is and the overwhelming willingness to move toward a goal oriented recovery. Constantly redefining performance objectives as he had done throughout his professional career is now helping him to define what is possible on his quest for a better quality of life. Bonne chance avec tout a venire!

Claudine Lanoix CHT
Centre Hyperbare De L'Ile,
Pincourt, Quebec

Thank you Michael Coss:

I have had the privilege of witnessing one of the most amazing comeback recoveries of any of my patients, and thanks to Michael and this book; he now shares his life's journey with the rest of the world. This is a touching story to the hearts of anyone who reads this book and even more important, has the ability to change the way you look at life. He does this by sharing with us his amazing and inspirational journey of a person that is committed to recovering from an unimaginable injury. Even worse was that medical specialists gave him no hope.

Michael starts off by giving us an idea of his life and family before an event that changes the life as he knew it. After suffering an intensive motor vehicle accident that put him into a vegetative comatose state, Michael Coss ha a choice; live with this debilitated condition and learn how to cope or take 2 steps forward and make a full recovery. Michael chose the latter and here begins his struggle and road to recovery. No one says it's easy and for Michael it was pure determination and courage. His attitude is what really sets him apart and I can honestly say, in all my 12 years of clinical practice and seeing patients I have but one thing to say: There is one major commonality among my patients who have made dramatic success, whether from a stroke, head injury, or cancer, and that is their attitude. Anyone who is suffering from any type of debilitating condition must read this book to see the attitude that Michael had throughout his difficult journey. This is an excellent read for giving anyone the motivation to overcome a serious health challenge. Where most people would stop, Michael keeps moving forward and eventually, I am convinced, he will achieve his dreams, his hopes, his ambitions and of course his ultimate goal; a goal that is a primary driving passion for Michael.

Dr. Zayd Ratansi, ND
Medical Director
Advanced Hyperbaric Centre
Coquitlam, BC

Introduction

Chances are you know someone with a traumatic brain injury (TBI). You may not even know they have it. It is, however, a fairly common injury. Though the symptoms are varied and the side effects can be hidden, it can be a tremendously challenging injury for survivors to manage.

I can say this with some confidence because I know the statistics. You see, I too suffer from a traumatic brain injury.

However, I'm one of the lucky ones.

Many people who suffer from traumatic brain injuries aren't so lucky.

What is a Traumatic Brain Injury?

A traumatic brain injury is a trauma to the brain. It can be caused by an impact—like a fall or being hit by something—or by a loss of oxygen to the brain. For example, drowning victims often suffer from TBI. It can also be caused by an intrusion. For example, a gunshot wound to the brain or a surgery can cause a traumatic brain injury.

When most people think about brain injuries, they imagine the loss of motor functions. This is true in many cases. Sometimes people are unable to walk, talk or move their body the way they used to. However, side effects of TBI are not always visible.

Many times the side effects are hidden. The results are often emotional changes, memory or cognitive changes, and the development of social anxieties or challenges.

If someone is recovering from mild TBI, also called a concussion or minor head injury, they may experience:

- Fatigue
- Headaches
- Visual disturbances
- Memory loss
- Poor attention/concentration
- Sleep disturbances
- Dizziness/loss of balance
- Irritability/emotional disturbances
- Feelings of depression
- Seizures

Mild traumatic brain injury is the most common type. However, it can still be quite serious and symptoms don't always show up right away. They may show up days or even weeks later.

A moderate brain injury is defined as an injury resulting in a loss of consciousness for longer than twenty minutes but less than six hours. These types of injuries are given a rating in the range of nine to twelve on the Glasgow Coma Scale. The Glasgow Coma Scale is a scoring system that's used to measure and record the level of consciousness after a brain injury.

A severe brain injury is defined as a brain injury resulting in a loss of consciousness for longer than six hours, and will receive a rating in the range of three to eight on the Glasgow Coma Scale. I scored an eight after my accident.

The side effects of a moderate to severe brain injury can include difficulties with:

- Attention
- Concentration
- Memory
- Processing speed

- Confusion
- Perseveration (the uncontrolled repetition of a response such as a phrase, word, or gesture)
- Impulsiveness
- Speech and language
- Vision difficulties
- Balance and motor skills
- Hearing difficulties or loss
- Diminished sense or loss of smell or taste
- Seizures
- Chronic pain
- Loss of digestive function
- Difficulty regulating body function
- Social-emotional changes like irritability and depression

As you can see, a person who suffers even mild to moderate TBI can have a very difficult road ahead of them. TBI changes lives.

Startling Facts About TBI

Because there is no TBI national registry, much of the data about traumatic brain injuries are estimated based on what the medical community actually does know. Many head injuries go unreported, meaning that the data can be skewed. However, the facts that we have are still quite shocking. Here's what we do know:

- According to the CDC, each year there are about two million people who sustain a traumatic brain injury in the U.S.
- About 52,000 people die from TBI in the U.S. each year—which accounts for 34% of all injury deaths. In Canada, more than 11,000 people die from TBI each year.
- Each year over 1.5 million Americans suffer nonfatal

traumatic brain injuries that do not require hospitalization. About the same number are reported to sustain a brain injury resulting in a loss of consciousness, but not severe enough to result in long-term institutionalization.

- Another 300,000 individuals suffer brain injuries each year severe enough to require hospitalization, with 99,000 of these injuries resulting in a lasting disability.
- According to Caregiver.org and other resources, an estimated 62.3 out of every 100,000 adults age fifteen and over are living with enduring functional impairments due to TBI. This statistic excludes most survivors of mild TBI.
- In Canada, brain injuries are the leading cause of death and disability for people under thirty-five years old.

Shocked yet? I bet you didn't know TBI was so common. Unfortunately, many people don't know about the various treatments available to help aid recovery. They also don't know how to prevent traumatic brain injuries.

Prevention

Interestingly, more males are affected by TBI than females. It may be simply related to the fact that they perform more "death defying" feats. For example, accidents that happen while participating in winter sports like skiing without a helmet, or riding a motorcycle without a helmet, are common causes. A simple football tackle gone wrong can cause a minor traumatic brain injury. A concussion is an instance of mild TBI.

Young people are also more at risk. Individuals aged fifteen to twenty-four have the highest risk of TBI. The risk also increases after age sixty.

My traumatic brain injury was the result of a car accident, a very common cause. In fact, motor vehicle accidents account for an estimated 28% of all traumatic brain injuries.

The Costs of TBI

According to the National Institute of Neurological Disorders and Stroke, the lifetime cost for one person surviving a severe TBI can reach $4 million. While many people focus on the direct financial costs of TBI—and these can be astronomically expensive—there are other significant costs that many people don't consider.

Personal relationships can suffer under the challenges of TBI. Imagine if a loved one suffered from TBI and their personality was forever changed. It happens and it can be difficult to recover from.

Continuing to have a relationship with that person may become difficult, as he or she is a different person after the injury. And that's only the beginning.

There are freedom costs too. Often a traumatic brain injury will result in the loss of a particular function. A person may have to relearn how to speak, be unable to walk, or lose memory function.

Many TBI sufferers are unable to return to work. In addition to a loss of income, this affects their self-worth, confidence and pride. In fact, depression is a common side effect of traumatic brain injuries.

According to a study published in the May 2010 issue of JAMA (Journal of the American Medical Association), "Major depressive disorder (MDD) may be the most common and disabling psychiatric condition in individuals with TBI. Poorer cognitive functioning, aggression and anxiety, greater functional disability, poorer recovery, higher rates of suicide attempts, and greater health care costs are thought to be associated with MDD after TBI."

This means that, even though a person may be recovering

physically from their injury, the emotional and mental recovery can take years. In fact, a person may never fully recover from their injury. As a person who has gone through a severe brain injury and years of ongoing recovery I can tell you one thing—the love and support of friends, family and caregivers matters.

It takes great courage to deal with the challenges TBI presents.

Treatment and Recovery: What Is Possible?

There are many different kinds of treatments available for patients of TBI. Often these treatments go hand in hand and work to support each other. My treatments have varied over time, each addressing a unique challenge.

Initially, one of the most powerful treatments I underwent was something called HBOT—Hyperbaric Oxygen Therapy. This treatment literally changed my life. I wouldn't be telling this story without it.

After a person enters the hospital and receives initial care for TBI, treatment can include rehabilitative care center treatment. This type of treatment helps a person learn to get back to daily life. If the injured survivor isn't ready for an independent living situation, then they may be sent to an acute treatment center. This type of center strives to offer life support and minimize and treat secondary injuries.

I have been residing in one of the Connect Communities homes for the last ten months and I strongly feel that all the employees and management are highly qualified to promote safe independent living as they treat me and others with the utmost quality care in a positive and very safe environment. I am gaining my independence again and what a wonderful feeling that is. I would highly recommend this organization to anyone looking to gain their independence again after suffering a similar injury.

Finally, some people may need to undergo surgical treatment.

This is usually designed to help improve blood flow and oxygen to the brain. They may also try to reduce swelling to prevent further brain damage.

How Can I Support Someone with TBI?

The road to recovery is long and bumpy. When I awoke from my coma, the only thing I could do was wiggle the thumb on my right hand. Today, several years later, I am learning to walk again, but my challenges are far from over. And I've had the kind of support, love and motivation that a person can only dream of. I'm truly blessed.

If you know someone with TBI, then I can only encourage you to provide him with as much love and support as you have to offer.

It takes great courage to keep going after a brain injury.

We TBI survivors ask that you treat us with dignity, respect and love. Not every day will be a good day. We rely on your advice, motivation and honesty. Clear communication is essential. Don't mislead a person struggling to recover from TBI. Tell him the truth. With your love and support, he can handle it!

Encourage TBI survivors to challenge themselves, to take risks and set aside fear. They've lived through an ordeal and have come out on the other side. The road, while it may be difficult and really bumpy, gets better. With your help, they can persevere.

This of course brings me to the purpose of this book and why I wanted to write "The Courage to Come Back."

What's the Purpose of this Book?

While I rarely bite off more than I can chew (I might have a big mouth), there are many purposes for this book. It's my greatest desire that ultimately this book gives hope to survivors.

It's about more than simply telling my story. I wouldn't be here without the amazing treatments, technology and medical science breakthroughs. However, I also wouldn't have come as far as I have without the love and support of my friends and family. It takes great strength to recover and manage a traumatic brain injury. The goal of this book is to give survivors that strength and the hope to continue recovering.

The profits from the sales of this book will be re-directed to The Michael Coss Brain Injury Foundation, which improves the quality of life of a child by putting him or her through Hyperbaric Oxygen treatments.

I imagine that if this book affects one life for the better, if it helps one person struggling with TBI to persevere, then it's all worth it.

I also hope that this book gives strength and encouragement to loved ones of people dealing with TBI. You have a tough job. You have to be there to support and motivate your survivor. I hope this book inspires you!

Finally, I hope this book raises awareness for my foundation, The Michael Coss Brain Injury Foundation, and for HBOT therapy.

Hyperbaric Oxygen is often the last chance for TBI sufferers. It's my goal to increase awareness of this life-giving therapy and to help those who need it.

Throughout this book I am honored to share my story. I'm even more honored to share the notes and messages from my friends, family and the medical professionals who have changed my life.

Thank you for this blessed opportunity!

CHAPTER ONE

On Cloud Nine

*Everything can be taken away from a man
but one thing: the last of human freedoms—
to choose one's attitude in any given set of
circumstances; to choose one's own way.*
-Victor Frank

It's amazing how quickly life can change.

Many people go through their lives without any struggles or challenges. Some suffer greatly. Others are faced with seemingly insurmountable challenges and come out on the other side successfully.

Who are the lucky ones?

I suppose that answer depends on whom you ask. I can tell you that what I appreciated about my life before my accident, and what I now appreciate, has changed in many ways.

You Know When You've Got it Good

I'll be the first to admit that before my accident I really did have it all. I had a beautiful wife who I loved very much. We were solid and building our dream life together.

I had two beautiful new babies. There's little that compares with being a new father.

I also had a job that I loved. Really! Who wouldn't love working for a beer company? And Molson Coors Canada is a great company.

I also had great friends, a supportive and close-knit family, and an active and fun life. Oh, and I had a new home, too, one that fit my lifestyle and growing family.

Life was darned near perfect.

Yep. I had it all, and on the day of my accident I knew it—I was on cloud nine.

I don't want to bore you with too many details. However, much about my life before my accident had a direct effect on my recovery. My family, friends and even my childhood experiences all helped create a person who had the courage to come back.

I'm sharing this personal information with you in the hope that you may see some of the same experiences in yourself. May my experiences help you persevere and find hope. May my experiences help you support other traumatic brain injury survivors live the best lives possible.

The Coss Clan and Beyond

Raised to embrace life, I had a typical family in many ways. What's typical of them is the way they've changed their life to help me recover and get back on my feet (quite literally).

I spent my early teenage years growing up in Newmarket, Ontario. It's a small town in southern Ontario, about thirty miles north of Toronto. It had a population of around 25,000 when I was there. It was certainly not a booming metropolis, but I think the atmosphere was great for growing up.

I have always been a competitive person and I believe my parents helped instill that in me. They encouraged me and my siblings to follow our passions and interests—even when those interests were a bit risky.

I remember when my brother Brian was injured during our dirt bike "time trials." We were a little crazy on those bikes. Brian flew over the handlebars and fell face first, landing smack onto his chin.

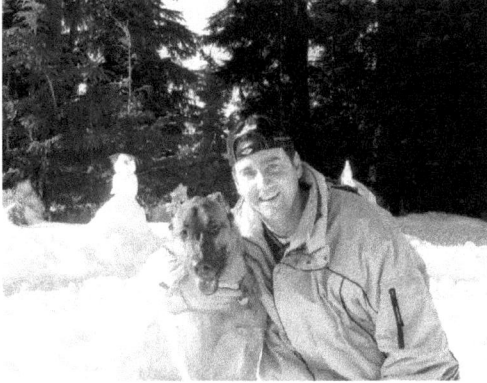

Michael and Murphy

We also used to take our German shepherd dog for a nice long walk in the farmer's fields right behind our house while we rode our dirt bikes.

I think in many ways our risk taking helped me as an adult. I certainly took many risks in my life. Some paid off. Some didn't.

However, as a TBI survivor you have to be willing to take risks. And some days just getting out of bed is a risk.

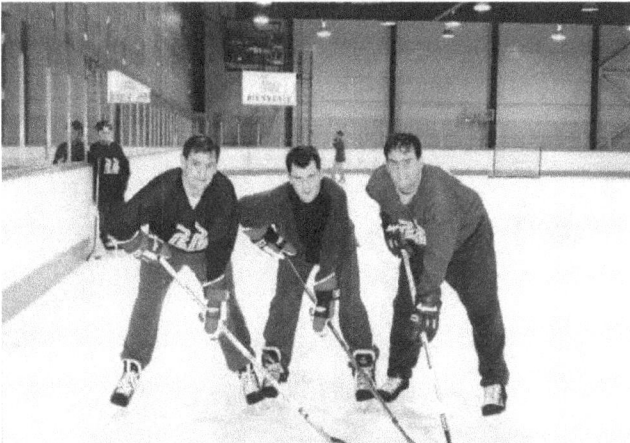

Hockey with brothers Brian & Dwayne

In addition to my recovery from TBI, competitiveness also played a role in my childhood ambitions. As an adolescent I played hockey. To this day I still love the sport! The highlight of my earlier years was when my hockey team won the all Ontario hockey championship. I was just twelve years old and I was one of the goaltenders on the "AA" hockey team.

I played other sports too, like soccer, baseball, and basketball. But my favorite by far was (and still is) ice hockey.

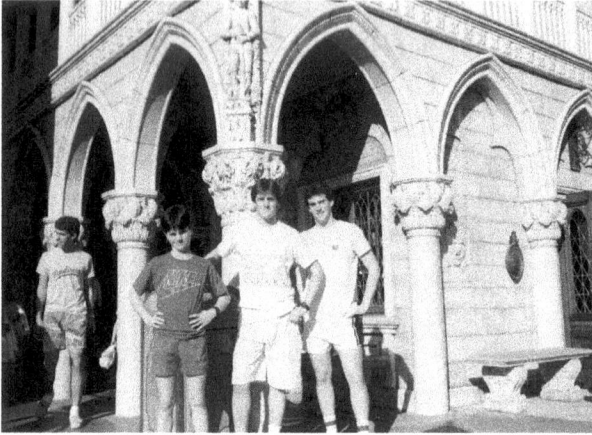

I have fond memories of my childhood and am sure they molded me into the man I am today, helping me to become the kind of person who could handle the challenges of TBI.

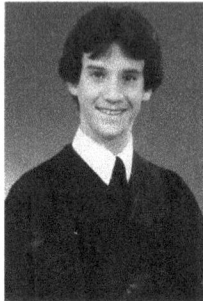

Michael's graduation

When I was a teenager we moved to Sainte-Foy, Quebec City, and I spent my last two years of high school there. I graduated from Katimavik High School in 1985. It was one of three English high schools in a French province.

One of my highlights from high school was when we took a bus trip to New York City and visited the Bronx. That kind of place sticks with you!

While I certainly kept busy looking at the ladies, I worked a lot too. I developed a hard work ethic as a teenager. As a young man, one of my very first jobs was as a cook at McDonald's. I also worked at Maryvale Farms for two Christian Brothers: Brother John and Brother Peter. There I performed odd jobs like mowing the lawn, painting, cleaning the house, and cooking. I still have some of my very first pay stubs!

I had several newspaper routes. I mowed the neighbors' lawns in the summertime and I shoveled their driveways in the wintertime for extra pocket money. I guess that I had a fairly normal upbringing. However, looking back I can see how my childhood and upbringing prepared me for the challenges ahead. My work ethic alone has helped me accomplish a lot over these past few years

Days after my accident, my parents permanently relocated from Quebec City to Vancouver, BC. They left family, friends and co-workers behind to be by my side. They were there through thick and thin to support my wife, my children, and me. A child cannot ask for more from their parents than what my parents have given me. They're amazing.

While I'm sure it's not a hardship to be closer to your grandchildren, my parents did give up a lot to move. My father was able to arrange a long distance relationship with his boss and work from our home in Vancouver. They also were able to trade in the snow of Quebec City and move to beautiful Vancouver, BC.

While I've always been grateful to my parents for all they've taught me and all they've given me, their move to Vancouver has further strengthened and solidified our relationship.

I am very fortunate and thankful as both my parents continue to improve my life and the life of my family.

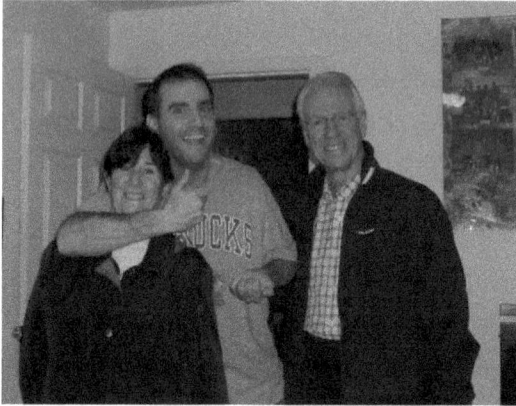

Michael and his parents, Suzette and Robert Coss

My cousin, Caroline Archer, shared this memory from our childhood and it's a perfect example of how close our family is.

"Out of all the cousins within the Coss family, our Christmas holidays were always spent in Lac Beauport with my brothers; Antho and Si and our cousins Mike, Brian and Dwayne. We were all close in age—thus the reason for the great camaraderie that developed within our growing years. The spirit of familiarity and closeness was soon to be discovered when we put on our snowsuits and winter gear and ventured into the deep snow that had still been untouched.

We would run up and down the hills in front of Pat and Linda's 'cottage' and throughout the many different cross-country skiing paths outback. Looking back…what a peaceful, serene and picturesque place that was. Well, maybe not so peaceful for me when the boys would decide to denote a touch of support and cooperativeness with one another and begin taunting me with challenging games such as face plants and snowball fights.

Their mocking smiles always gave it away and I knew I was in for a fight of my own in trying to get away from whatever they had up their sleeves. The leaders of the pack...who else but Mike and Antho? I can still hear their laughter bellying up out of their mouths with calculative defeat.

They worked with and fed off one another to chew over what they had done to their sister and cousin...their prey. To repaint those moments would certainly be a great joy. After hours of being outside, rosy cheeks and all, we would get ready for the festivities and great food the women had been laboring over all day.

Gathered around the table we would devour the best chicken potpie. The chicken potpie is still being served but the company has changed. On to creating new and wonderful memories."

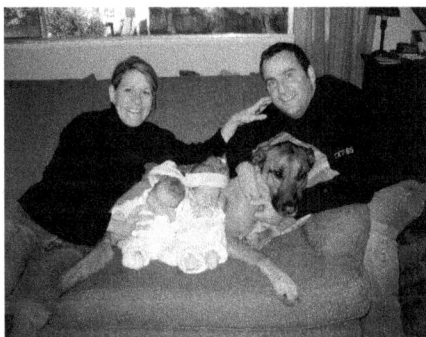

Ann, Michael & newborns Danielle & Nathan

My New Family: A Guy's Gotta Grow Up Sometime, Right?

I met my wife Ann about twelve years ago when I was a sales representative for JM Schneider Meats and she worked as a deli clerk for IGA grocery store. She's gorgeous and instantly caught my eye. Not one to hesitate, I made my moves.

We hit it off instantly. I was a licensed plane pilot at the time and took Ann on a scenic flight over the city of Vancouver and over the Rocky Mountains.

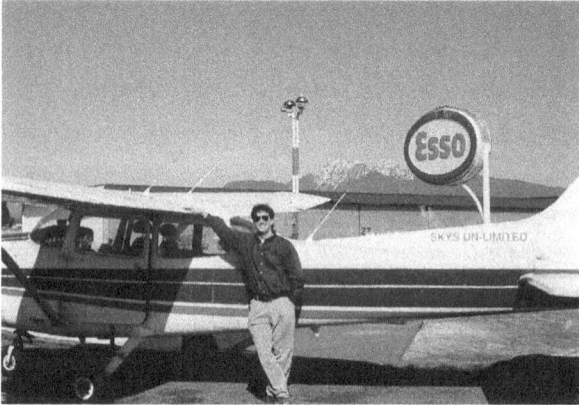

Michael the pilot

As you can imagine, I swept her off her feet! We moved in together shortly thereafter and got married.

Our wedding was a wonderful and memorable event. We wed in Nuevo Vallarta, Mexico, in front of fifty-five family members, friends, and co-workers at an all-inclusive resort called *Club Marival.* We wanted all our guests to also enjoy a nice vacation as well as witness and be a part of our wedding. Some of our guests swam in the swimming pools or the ocean. Some people went deep-sea fishing, snorkeling, ATV'ing, or simply shopping.

My best man, Wayne Farrell, was an old high school friend. At that time he was in the army and was stationed in Egypt. As a special thank you, Ann and I organized and hosted a sunset cruise for all our guests.

After the honeymoon, we purchased a one-bedroom condominium in a complex called The Kennedy, and we lived in it for a number of years. When we sold our condo unit, we purchased a half duplex as an entry level home and we stayed there for a few more years. Eventually, through a few investment decisions, we were about to purchase our current family home. Our dream home.

I'd have to say that I was on cloud nine just prior to my injury. I was living life in the fast lane. Ann and I found out that we were about to be new parents to not just one child, but twins. We'd been married for five years and felt very solid as a couple. We were both very much looking forward to being new parents.

Many things changed after my accident. Many things stayed the same. I still love my wife Ann with my whole heart and we have two beautiful children. They're the inspiration and the motivation that get me through the tough moments.

My Career: Climbing the Ladder

Prior to working for Molson Coors Canada, I worked for Rothman's Benson & Hedges for eight years. During my time there, I worked my way up. Again, that work ethic and competitive spirit took me far—I actually won the Salesman of the Year award while I was there.

Not really happy with the direction the cigarette industry was going in, I decided it was time to move on. In 1996, I was hired by Molson Coors Canada as a sales representative. Once again, I worked my way up. I worked the streets for five years before being offered my job within Field Marketing. It was a hard-earned dream come true.

The Field Marketing department is the department that designs, creates and builds the programs for the sales representatives so they can sell more beer than our competitors. I excelled as a sales representative and loved the job and the career I built. I made many solid and wonderful relationships.

I took my role seriously and I enjoyed representing Molson Coors Canada very much. But I had grown and I was ready for a new position within the organization. I was very competitive and that urge began to once again surface. I wanted to move up the ladder. Also, I was about to become a new father, so the change of position was very much welcomed by the Molson organization.

I'd earned the promotion six months before the accident. I have to say that my position as a sales representative allowed me to come out of my shell. I was able to further develop my communication, negotiation, and social confidence skills.

This most certainly helped me become the person I am today. It has helped me find the courage to continue my recovery. It's helped me start a charitable foundation. And ultimately it helped me decide to write this book.

I miss my job and especially the people that I work with.

My closest co-workers were Heath Lefroy, David Riggs, Greg Hutchings and Darren Opsahl. I was also quite close to Kerri Gama, our sales administrator.

I would like to acknowledge and thank the person who hired me, Ronnie Paterson. He was a great mentor and teacher to me. He was also a bit of a father figure to me. I aspire to be the kind of man and father he is to his wife and children. He is definitely a role model for me. His favorite saying is "one more then the bill."

He used to own a pub located in White Rock called Hampton's where he hosted many fundraisers for my family and me. He has two sons, Tyler and Troy.

Troy has been chosen to play for the Richmond Sockeyes. Ronnie played goal for Canadian Olympic Team back in 1980. He has numerous contacts and a vast circle of friends. I would definitely go to bat for RP and so would many other people.

He is in the process of opening up a brand new pub and beer and wine store. I want to wish Ronnie and his family nothing but success with his new business venture. I'm sure I'll be hoisting one up in the very near future with him.

One big promotion or event that I organized was watching a Vancouver Canucks game at Samz pub in Langley with a few of my coworkers and Dan Cloutier, who played goal for the Vancouver

Canucks. As a sales rep for Molson Coors Canada, I called both on retail accounts like beer & wine stores, government liquor stores, and on-premise accounts (which were the pubs).

We had great sales administrators like Kerri Gama and Darcie Prokop. They both played a key role within our organization by maintaining our budgets to make sure we stayed between the pipes, just like a goaltender on a hockey team.

Our department was run by Tim Cowley, or as he was known, "Crusher." He was a sales rep on the streets like I was. I am glad that I was on the same side of the fence as Tim and didn't have to call up against him.

Our department consisted of Matt Johnson, myself, and Tim as our boss. It has since grown and includes Denise Kerr, who used to be our sales rep in Whistler, and Craig DiRocco, who was a retail rep. We've had quite a few changes and additions to the team since my accident.

My Health: Poster Boy for Molson Canadian

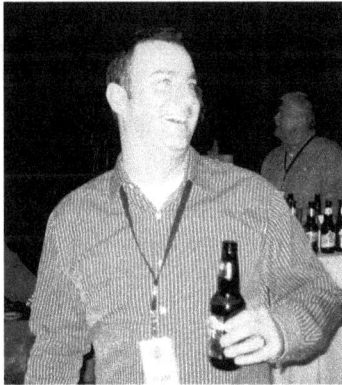

If you saw me now, you'd never imagine that I used to be the poster boy for Molson Canadian!

I weighed 210 lbs and was in decent shape. I played softball, golf, and hockey and lived an active, albeit not as healthy as I could have been, lifestyle.

I mean, it's tough to be really healthy when you sample beer and tour pubs for a living. And clients don't like to be wooed over broccoli. Suffice it to say that I was well-fed and spent a good amount of my time in pubs.

Prior to my injury, I belonged to a slow-pitch softball team called the Bad News Beers. Fun name, right? It was a great time full of memorable friends and road trips.

There's no slow-pitch softball in my life right anymore. At least not as a participant. But in many ways I am much healthier than I used to be. Today I weigh 153 pounds and my diet is significantly healthier.

You wouldn't imagine that recovering from TBI would make me healthier, but it has. When you're focused on your body and striving to improve and get stronger, everything you put into it matters.

My Goals: Some Change, Some Stay the Same

Once upon a time, my goals were the same as those of most folks. I wanted to continue climbing the ladder at my company. I wanted to expand my family. I wanted to have fun, love a lot, and live life to its fullest. I wanted to raise beautiful, strong and happy children and make a difference in the world.

Since my accident, not much of that has really changed. I still want to have fun, love a lot, and live life to its fullest. I still want to raise beautiful, strong and happy children. And I still want to make a difference in the world.

It's just that now my approach is different. Now my challenges and goals are focused on helping others recover from traumatic brain injury. I want to inspire and motivate. I want to remind others who are suffering, frustrated or discouraged about how amazing life can be.

However, I also want to walk freely and hold my children's hands.

There will be more challenges along the way. After five years of recovery from that fateful accident, I know that to be true. Life is full of challenges.

Some days will be discouraging. However, I also know that I've come a long way. I have a bright future ahead of me. I have wonderful parents, friends and caregivers. I have wonderful friends, a supportive family and two beautiful children.

Life is good!

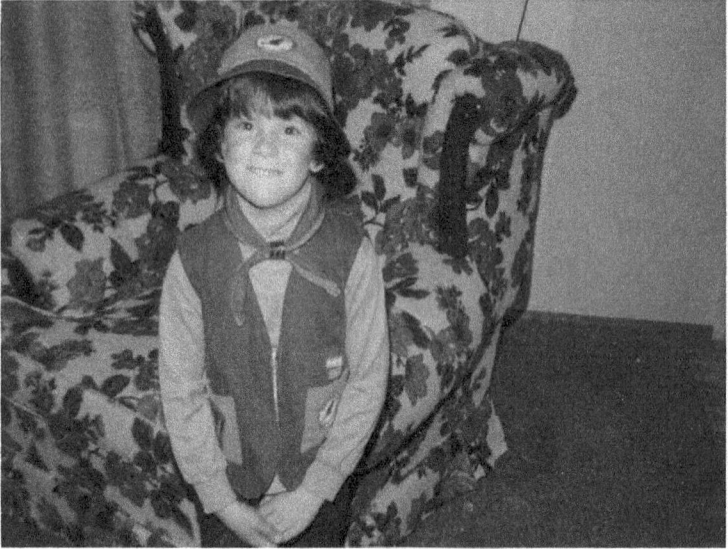

Michael at five years old

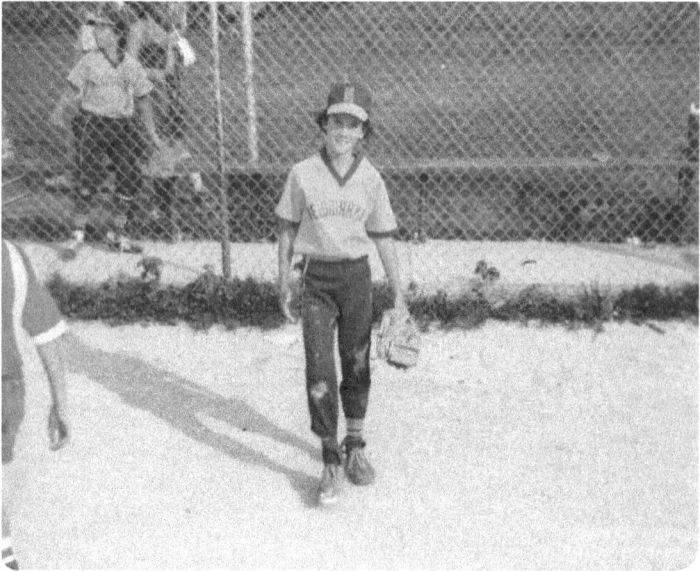

Michael at age eleven playing baseball

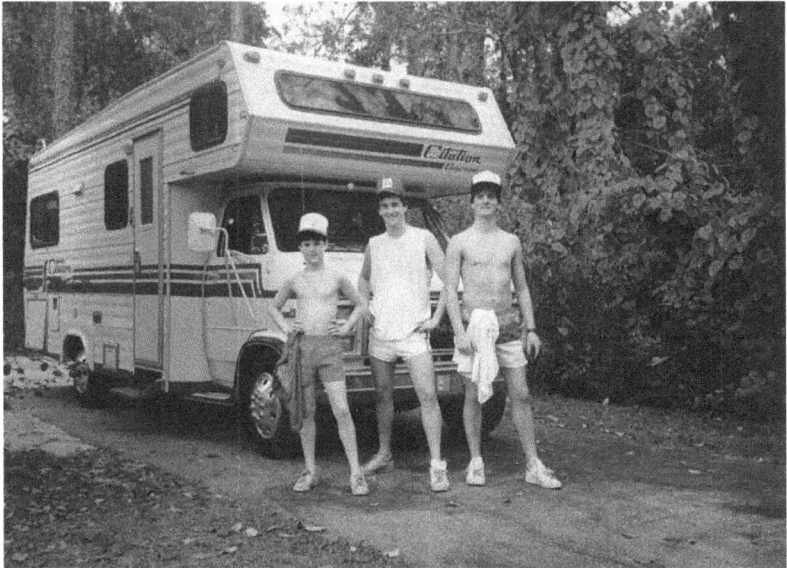

Christmas in Florida with Brian & Dwayne

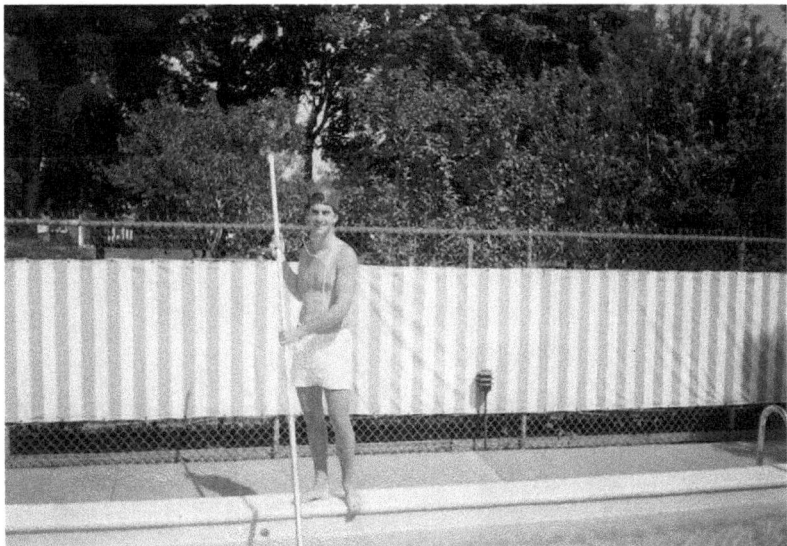

Michael at age fifteen

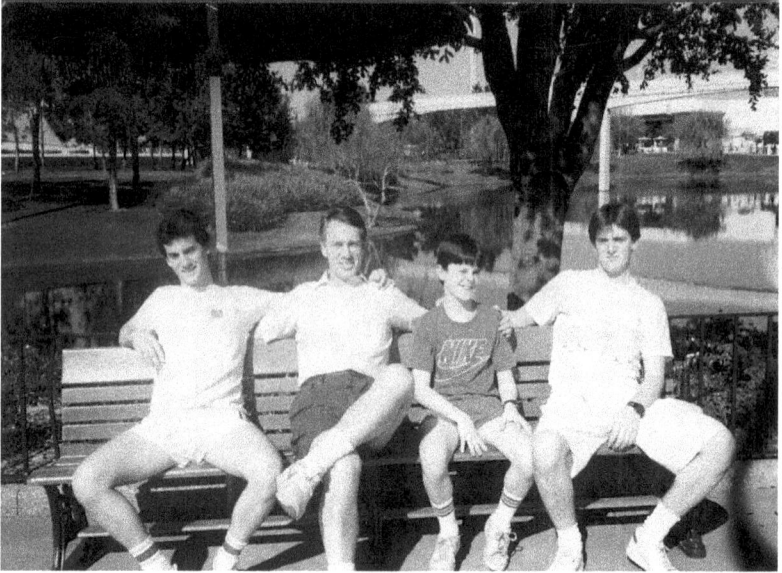

Christmas vacation in Florida

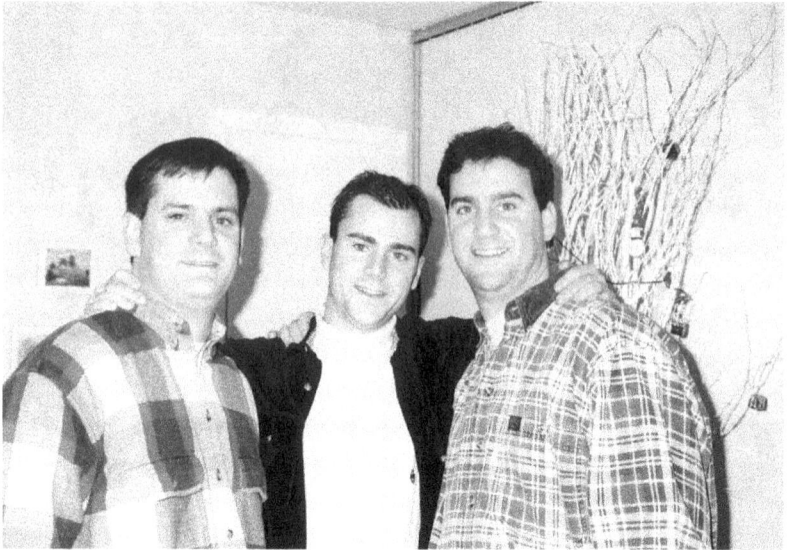

Michael with brothers Dwayne & Brian

~Personal Essays~

Because there are layers to a person's life and because others can sometimes tell the story better, I'd like to share stories and essays written by friends, family and healthcare providers throughout this book. At the end of each chapter I've included a few that are relevant to the chapter's material.

And because so many wonderful people have shared so much, the entire last chapter is a collection of essays and stories. I wouldn't be here without the amazing grace and support of the people in my life.

It's my honor to share their stories with you.

My name is Don Davis.

I met Mike in 1993, a few weeks after I got promoted to District Sales Manager at Rothmans, Benson & Hedges Inc. In fact, I hired Mike to replace the sales position that I had just been promoted from. Michael worked for me for most of the eight years he was at RBH. It was a sad day for both RBH and me when he decided to leave. I have a couple of short stories to share with all of you that will explain what type of person Michael is.

When I was going through the interview process with Mike, he purposely did not inform us that his father is working for RBH in Quebec. In fact, it was one of our long-term administrative staff employees that recognized the last name and phoned our HQ in Toronto to check on this. We were told that there is a Bob Coss working as a Supervisor in our Quebec City plant and that he has 3 sons one of them named Michael. The day that I was hiring Mike, I asked him if this was his father and why did he not reveal the fact that his father is working for RBH?

His answer was what I would expect from Michael, "I wanted to get the job on my own merit ".

My second story is a few years later when Michael won our Salesman of the Year award for Western Canada. The rest of Michael's family lived on the East coast and the award ceremony was to be at our National Sales conference in Montreal. As the winner of this award is a secret until the actual ceremony, I went to our Director to tell him that it would be a great moment if Bob Coss could be there to witness his son win such a prestigious company award. The arrangements were made and the result was a great moment to watch for everyone, a moment in time for a father and son.

So you ask what word I would use to describe Michael............ PROUD!!!!!

Proud of his accomplishments, his family and the friends he is surrounded by.

Hey Mike hopes this works for you; I can still see you and your father embracing on that stage.... what a moment!!

Regards, your friend, Don.

Mikey!

I associate Mike with anything that is fun and filled with laughter. He's the life of the party, and the one to always reassure you with a quick yet warm smile.

A dedicated business man, family man, and friend. His perseverance is remarkable and his positive attitude throughout his life has inspired and touched all who have come in contact with him.

I met Mike in 1994 when he started dating my cousin Annie. I in fact was the one who encouraged Annie to accept Mike's invitation to a date, when she was still unsure herself. (Not because Mike wasn't a friendly, hot sales guy for Schneider's!) Eventually they hooked up and the rest is history!

I love Mike and consider him more of a brother than a friend or relative by marriage. He has always been the best uncle to Jacob and Makenna and they ask for him often. He is a special man who will always hold a huge chunk of my heart and my family's.

Koreen Carl

Mike Coss—"Top Gun" Sales Rep Molson Brewery

I have known Mike, both from my days as a Brand Manager at Molson Breweries and later when I worked at Heineken Canada and Mike represented the Heineken brand on behalf of the distributor at Molson.

Mike was well known as one of the top Molson on-premise sales reps on the BC sales team and if you were a top priority account, you could be sure Mike did an excellent job of "taking care of business." I think it was because of his earlier experience as a cigarette sales rep, but Mike was very disciplined in terms of his call patterns and was a strong proponent of "promising less and deliver more." Mike's promotions were always very well received by both customers and consumers and usually included many special extras.

An example of Mike's dedication was Hampton's Pub, which was the #1 Heineken volume draught account for many years. This may surprise some people, as it is not the biggest or highest profile pub in the market. However the Heineken brand was extremely well supported by the rep and the ownership embraced the concept of offering higher margin products to their consumers. Furthermore, the delivery of the "tap to table" experience was well executed by the wait staff and each year there were a number of special promotions such as "Win a Heineken fridge" contests that captured the imagination of the consumer and increased sales year over year. Simple but effective when executed well!

It was unfortunate that Mike and Ronnie both chose to be goaltenders as it truly impacted our relationship. Although we each considered ourselves students of the game of hockey…we must have gone to different classes!

Continued

Over a beer we would often discuss the intricacies of the game and what was happening with our Canucks. However as a defenseman; as much as I tried to explain what was really happening out on the ice…They just didn't seem to get it. In the end for or Mike it all came down to "Bleu Blanc et Rouge" and for Ronnie it was all about those crazy Leafs.

Although Mike had moved on to a new position as Assistant Field Marketing manager, I first heard of Mike's accident within an hour through a phone call from Ron Paterson, which indicates how close they were as friends. I often think about Mike's accident as I was also a rep and manager spending many hours, especially in my early working years putting in many miles to visit a new account or to organize another promotion on behalf of Molson.

People are always quick to note the fun side of being a "beer rep" but it takes a special dedication to go the extra mile to be a great beer rep. I believe Mike's many licensee contacts and supporters are an indication of the level of appreciation Mike has earned over the course of his career.

Bruce Brill

CHAPTER TWO

That Fateful Day

My daily Thoughts and Commitments:
"All things are possible when you believe."
"Man becomes what he thinks about."
"Laughter attracts joy, releases negativity, and leads to miraculous cures."
"I focus on my full recovery."

Most people imagine that car accidents are either due to bad weather or someone else's negligence.

While this is true in many cases, sometimes accidents just happen.

I have to be a hundred percent upfront here and let you know that I don't remember the accident. This is common with car accident survivors and those who experience traumatic brain injury. 28% of traumatic brain injury incidents are the result of car accidents.

There are many theories as to why people don't remember their accident. I imagine that not remembering is a protective mechanism because our bodies are so good at keeping us alive. We don't remember because it's better not to. My brain needed to focus on more important activities than memory. It needed to

23

protect itself and stay alive.

I don't mind not remembering. It's not important. Today is important. Now. Tomorrow. The past cannot be changed. But I can share it with you as others told it to me.

That Fateful Day

May 18th, 2006.

The weather was picture perfect. Not a gust of wind or a drop of rain in sight. In fact, with the sun high in the sky it would have been a perfect day for a picnic in the park. As it was, we were headed to Kelowna, British Columbia.

We were on our way to a work event. It was a golf tournament hosted by Maxim. I'd been in my new position at Molson for a few months and it was going well. I loved my new job and the perk of this golf event was a highlight. I was looking forward to visiting my best friend, too.

We were going to be staying with Jay Heer and his wife, Jodi. They lived in beautiful Kelowna and also had two children. I hadn't seen him for a while and was really looking forward to spending some time with Jay and his family.

Jay and I had developed a strong friendship when we worked for the tobacco company, Rothmans, Benson & Hedges as sales representatives prior to moving on to Molson Coors Canada. We had similar interests—we played the same position in ice hockey (goalie) and we were both extremely competitive. We had sales as a similar interest and passion, and we both hated to lose, whether it was in ice hockey or sales.

We also enjoyed following and watching another sport—the NFL. We made the trip down to Seattle, Washington, to watch several games of the Seattle Seahawks. When Jay joined Molson Coors Canada as a sales representative in Kelowna, we played ice hockey at opposite ends of the ice as goaltenders. We played a few times at General Motors Place, now known as Rogers Arena, at opposite ends of the ice with our co-workers and customers as well.

Excited for the day ahead, I'd piled my wife and two six-month-old children in our van. It is about a 200 mile drive, give or take a few miles, so we got an early start and were on the road by nine in the morning.

Somewhere along the way, along the Coquihalla Highway, notably one of the most beautiful highways in the country, an animal ran out in front of my vehicle. Again, this isn't something I remember. It is supposition. Wildlife is common along the Coquihalla. It passes through some of the most beautiful landscapes in the province. It's both a fast route between Vancouver and Kelowna, but also a common scenic drive.

Just outside of Merritt, I swerved to avoid the animal. My car left the road. Many cars don't have the ability to combat the physics of a quick change in direction. My minivan was no different. It rolled.

Experts at accident re-creation estimate that it rolled at least one and a half times. It's possible that the car rolled more, and at the speed we were traveling it's quite likely. My brother saw the vehicle after the accident and said he was shocked we walked away from it.

I am thankful for many things about that day, but two things stand out:

1. No other cars were involved in the accident. It was classified as a single car rollover.
2. My wife and children survived. If they hadn't, my story would be very different.

My wife, Ann, broke her wrist. Danielle, my little six month old daughter managed to escape uninjured save a bloody nose. My son, Nathan, wasn't so lucky. He suffered a fractured skull. I can only imagine what Ann went through that day. Doctors induced little Nathan into a coma. He stayed in that coma for ten days.

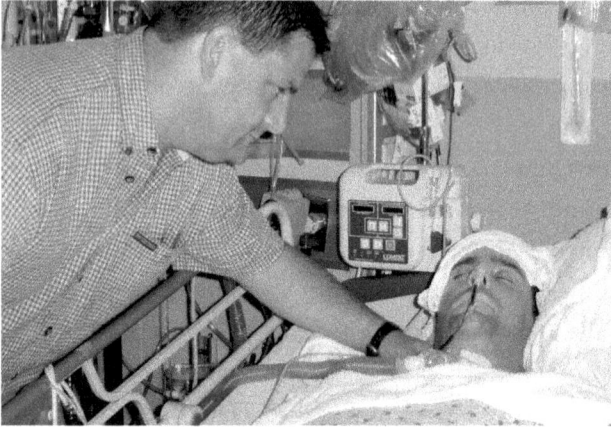

As you know, I suffered a traumatic brain injury. The diagnosis was diffuse axonal brain injury.

Diffuse axonal injury is not the result of hitting your head against something. It's what happens when your brain essentially bounces around inside your skull. It's one of the most common types of brain injuries. It's also one of the most devastating. It results in widespread damage, with many injured areas on the brain. The result is often unconsciousness, coma, and a persistent vegetative state.

According to gathered statistics, the result of DAI is often coma. Over 90% of patients with severe DAI never regain. Those who do wake up often remain significantly impaired.

I fell into a deep coma. My coma ranked an eight on the Glasgow Coma Scale. The Glasgow Coma Scale is ranked on a point system from one to fifteen.

The test measures the motor response, verbal response, and eye opening response with these values:

I. Motor Response

6 - Obeys commands fully
5 - Localizes to noxious stimuli
4 - Withdraws from noxious stimuli
3 - Abnormal flexion, i.e. decorticate posturing
2 - Extensor response, i.e. decerebrate posturing
1 - No response

II. Verbal Response

5 - Alert and Oriented
4 - Confused, yet coherent, speech
3 - Inappropriate words and jumbled phrases consisting of words
2 - Incomprehensible sounds
1 - No sounds

III. Eye Opening

4 - Spontaneous eye opening
3 - Eyes open to speech
2 - Eyes open to pain
1 - No eye opening

The final score is determined by adding the values of from each of the three main categories.

This number helps medical practitioners categorize the four possible levels for survival, with a lower number indicating a more severe injury and a poorer prognosis:

Moderate Disability (9-12):

• Loss of consciousness greater than 30 minutes.
• Physical or cognitive impairments that may or may not be

resolved.
- Benefits from rehabilitation.

Severe Disability (3-8):

- Coma: unconscious state.
- No meaningful response, no voluntary activities.

Vegetative State (Less Than 3):

- Sleep/wake cycles.
- Arousal, but no interaction with environment.
- No localized response to pain.

Persistent Vegetative State:

- Vegetative state lasting longer than one month.

Brain Death:

- No brain function.
- Specific criteria needed for making this diagnosis.

(Information based on Glasgow Coma Scale at TraumaticBrainInjury.com)

I scored eight points and remained curled up in the fetal position and in a coma for the next six and a half months.

The Next Few Days

For the first two weeks after the accident I was cared for in the Royal Inland Hospital in Kamloops. There, they tended to my care, kept me alive, and tried to rouse me from my coma. My parents sat by my bedside during the day. My brother Dwayne and his wife Chantelle sat by my bedside at night. My wife, as you might expect, sat by Nathan's bedside. It was a dark time for all.

As I think about their love and devotion right now it brings me to tears. Their presence at my side means the world to me. Such love, faith, and devotion. That's the power of a family. I would do anything for my family and I know they would do anything for me. They've shown this to be true.

Imagine sitting at the bedside of a family member. You don't know if he is going to make it. And even if he does, you wonder what the future has in store for him. All you want for your children is for them to live happy and fulfilling lives. It seems sometimes, this isn't possible. When something like this happens you wonder if they're going to make it, if they're going to get to live the life you want them to.

Being a father, I cannot imagine being in the position my parents were in. It has to have been an agonizing experience. Yet, at the same time it is my wish that everyone who experiences trauma have the same support.

My in-laws were there to help Ann in any way they could. Household tasks and childcare don't seem like much until you are forced to handle everything and care for a child and husband in the hospital. My in-laws helped prepare meals, take the dog for walks, take care of daily household chores, babysit and support Ann thorough the entire ordeal.

My parents promptly relocated to Vancouver from Quebec City. In fact, they made this life change the day after my injury. They left family members, friends, and co-workers behind. Their decisions and actions over the next six and a half months changed my life.

On May 30th, a little less than a month after the accident, I was transferred by air ambulance to Royal Columbian Hospital in New Westminster. My mother accompanied me in the ambulance. The doctors at Kamloops were unable to care for a long-term coma patient and the Royal Columbian was better equipped to meet my long-term care needs. Doctors told my parents and family that the fact that I was young was a positive sign, but that it would be a long road to recovery and they should pray for a miracle.

I then spent the next six months at Royal Columbian before moving to Eagle Ridge Hospital in December.

CHAPTER THREE

Time Flies When You're Having Fun

*"Time is free, but it's priceless. You can't
own it, but you can use it. You can't keep
it, but you can spend it. Once you've lost it
you can never get it back."*
-Harvey MacKay

You wouldn't think you'd miss much when you're asleep for
six and a half months, but a lot can change. This is especially true
when it comes to children. They learn and grow so very quickly.

I was in a coma for more than six months. In that amount of
time, a baby learns to say a few words.

They take their first steps. They grow, they laugh. They cry.

I missed that precious time with my children. I'll never get
it back. I missed all those late night feedings with Ann. I missed
sharing those treasured moments of new parenting. Yet, I'm
grateful, so grateful!

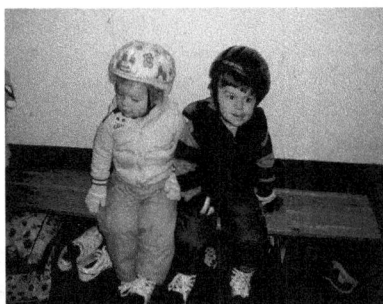

I could have missed so much more.

During the time I was away, here are just some of the events that occurred:

- April 8th: In an incident known as the Shedden massacre, the bodies of eight men, all shot to death, were found in a field in Ontario, Canada. Their murders were linked to the Bandidos motorcycle gang.

- April 22nd: Four Canadian soldiers were killed 75 kilometers north of Kandahar, Afghanistan by a roadside bomb planted by Taliban militants. It was the worst single day combat loss for the Canadian army since the Korean War.

- May 21st: The Swedish ice hockey team Tre Kronor took gold in the World Championship, becoming the first nation to hold both the World and Olympic titles in the same year.

- May 26th: The May 2006 Java earthquake killed over 5,700 people, and left 200,000 homeless.

- May 27th: The May 2006 Java earthquake struck again, devastating Bantul and the city of Yogyakarta, killing over 6,600 people.

- June 21st: Pluto's newly discovered moons were officially named Nix and Hydra.

- June 25th: The U.S.'s second richest man, Warren Buffet, announced that he will donate over $30 billion to the foundation started by the richest man, Bill Gates.

- July 4th: North Korea tests four short-range missiles, one medium-range missile, and a long-range Taepodong-2.

- July 30th: The world's longest running music show, Top of the Pops, is broadcast for the last time on BBC Two. The show had aired for forty-two years.

- July 31st: Fidel Castro temporarily handed over power to brother Raúl Castro. This led to a celebration in Little Havana Miami, Florida, in which many Cuban Americans participated.

- August 10th: Scotland Yard uncovered a serious terrorist plot to destroy aircraft travelling from the United Kingdom to the United States. All toiletries were banned from commercial airplanes. This of course has caused a number of hassles for travelers and was the beginning of travel headaches in North America and beyond. Still, it's better to be safe.

- August 24th: The International Astronomical Union (IAU) redefined the term "planet" such that Pluto is now considered a Dwarf Planet.

- August 31st: Stolen on August 22, 2004, Edvard Munch's famous painting The Scream was recovered in a raid by Norwegian police.

- September 12th: With its release of iTunes 7, Apple announces that people have bought over 1.5 billion songs in three years.

- October 9th: North Korea allegedly tested its first nuclear device.

- October 17th: The United States population reached 300 million.

- October 24th: Justice Rutherford of the Ontario Superior Court of Justice struck down the "motive clause," an important part of the Canadian Anti-Terrorism Act.

- November 27th: The Canadian House of Commons endorsed Prime Minister Stephen Harper's motion to declare Québécois a nation within a unified Canada.

- December 6th: NASA revealed photographs taken by Mars Global Surveyor that suggested the presence of liquid water on Mars.

(HistoryOrb.com helped me uncover much of this information.)

All of this seems so significant and insignificant at the same time. Yet nothing is more important than the fact that while I was away, my body stayed alive. It continued to heal. It fought to survive.

When medical services arrived at the scene of the accident, I was in a comatose state. Consequently, I was airlifted to Kamloops Royal Inland Hospital where my body was assessed by neurosurgery and had shunts inserted. Despite the best efforts of the staff there, I remained comatose.

Two weeks later, I was transferred to Royal Columbian Hospital, in part to be closer to my family. I was in the critical care unit, then the neurology unit. All the time, I was unable to follow commands. My injuries were nearly fatal. Despite comprehensive treatment at two hospitals, I remained in a coma for six and half months.

Amazing Ann

Ann, my wife, was nothing short of amazing. Raising twin babies isn't easy. Raising them by yourself is a feat. It takes a strong, brave and determined person. That's Ann.

She has spent the past five years raising them on her own, while I've been recovering from my accident.

Hats off to her, with a huge round of applause!

Even with the support of my wonderful parents and in-laws, she has her hands full. She's bearing a responsibility that would bring many people to their knees.

During my recovery, my parents and in-laws helped. They assisted with all the tasks required to manage and maintain a household. They mowed the lawn, helped with repairs. They also babysat, prepared meals, and helped Ann in any way they could.

I'll be indebted to them for the rest of my life. I'm sure it was a long couple of months!

Fast Forward Three Months

After a few months in a deep coma, many doctors begin to lose hope. That was the case for me. Often, if your body doesn't pull out of a coma naturally within a few weeks, you'll remain in a vegetative state. One doctor told my father that there was nothing that could be done for me, that I'd have to be put in a permanent facility for the rest of my life.

Another doctor told my father that it would take a miracle.

If That's What it Takes...

My parents are fighters. They don't give up hope and they don't take no for an answer. They began researching online for answers. They found it in the form of hyperbaric oxygen therapy, or HBOT. It's a treatment that pumps oxygen into the body at a higher level than atmospheric pressure. It's not approved by Health Canada and it isn't covered by insurance. Still, the science behind the therapy makes sense.

At $125 per session, it was going to be an expensive experiment. But I suppose it's nothing that most parents wouldn't do for their child. With the help of friends, family, and my former co-workers at Molson Coors Canada, they raised the funds to proceed. The rest is history.

CHAPTER FOUR

The Awakening

The fact is, that to do anything in the world worth doing, we must not stand back shivering and thinking of the cold and danger, but jump in and scramble through as well as we can.
-Robert Cushing

What is a person to do when doctors say there is no hope? There are only two choices:

Give up

Or

Fight

My parents are fighters. The entire Coss clan is, really. It's both an endearing and probably frustrating trait!

Rather than give up, my family started digging for answers. They found some. Or rather my brother Dwayne did. He found HBOT and sent the information to my father.

HBOT is Hyperbaric Oxygen Therapy. There was substantial research supporting HBOT as a viable solution to my problem. My dad had found his hope. The hope some doctors said didn't exist.

A Little HBOT Education

The wonderful people over at the Advanced Hyperbaric and Recovery Center have created a website: www.hyperbaricexperts. com.

On the website you can download a free report about Hyperbaric treatments. The report covers a wealth of information, including research and case studies on hyperbaric oxygen therapy.

I've provided a description, with the help of information found in the free report "The Injured Brain Can Be Repaired," to help explain what HBOT is and why it's truly a miracle.

> If the brain is one of the highest consumers of oxygen (25% of oxygen in the body is used up by the brain), then it stands to reason that hyperbaric technology could be crucial in curing a brain disorder.
>
> In a normal setting, breathing 100% oxygen (as opposed to 21% oxygen in air) does not make a real difference in the oxygen that goes into the blood stream. When the blood goes to the lungs to get oxygen, the red blood cells can only carry so much and leave the lungs around 97% full. Note that even the little oxygen found in the air that you breathe is still not fully used up in this process.
>
> In a hyperbaric environment, the pressure alone forces the extra oxygen to be dissolved into the plasma (the fluid that carries the red blood cells). When oxygen gets into the blood, it is dissolved into two areas: the red blood cells and the blood plasma. In a hyperbaric chamber, you can breathe air, which is 21% oxygen, or you can breathe 100% oxygen. Either way, you are not only significantly increasing your blood oxygen levels, but also you are taking it one step further. You are getting the oxygen to areas that your red blood cells and your body can't get to because of the size of the red blood cells.
>
> In a hyperbaric environment, the oxygen that you breathe supersaturates above and beyond your red blood cell carrying capacity, and spills into the fluids that carry the red blood cells. The increased pressure, combined with the increased percentage of oxygen, will cause a net increase in the oxygen content.

The brain is one of the most unique organs that we have. It is basically submersed and bathed in fluid. This fluid is called cerebrospinal fluid, or CSF. As its name indicates, it bathes not only the brain, but also the spinal cord and every one of the nerves that come out of it.

So, if hyperbaric oxygen causes a significant rise in oxygen in body fluids, and we know that the brain is bathed by a body fluid known as cerebrospinal fluid, then it is easy to understand that a hyperbaric environment is absolutely crucial to the recovering brain that needs the extra oxygen for repair and regeneration. It is the only way to get a significant amount of oxygen into the brain.

So pressure, whether it is 1.3 ATA absolute or 3.0 ATA absolute, will significantly increase the oxygen in the body, more particularly the body fluids that red blood cells cannot deliver to, regardless of breathing 21% oxygen (normal air) or 100% oxygen (oxygen in a mask).

The bottom line is that if you have a brain injury, get yourself into a hyperbaric chamber. Whether you are breathing air or 100% oxygen, just get yourself into a chamber. The 'hyperbaric difference' will help allow you to 'soak up' the extra oxygen into your brain.

http://www.hyperbaricexperts.com/report/Free%20Brain%20Report-July%2024-09-FINAL.pdf

HBOT has been a miracle for helping survivors of Traumatic Brain Injury, like me. It also helps those who suffer from:
- Head Injury
- Autism
- Stroke
- Parkinson's Disease
- Alzheimer's Disease
- Multiple Sclerosis

- Huntington's Chorea
- Cerebral Palsy
- Fetal Alcohol Syndrome

As you can see, the research is convincing. My parents finally felt a surge of hope. HBOT seemed like it was my last chance for recovery.

A Wrinkle

While HBOT seemed to have real promise, there was a small problem.

It's really expensive.

It costs $125 per treatment. Patients often need a hundred or more treatments. And while it's an accepted treatment in many countries it isn't covered by Health Canada and insurance doesn't cover it. My family was on their own.

Once again the tough Coss family didn't give up hope. Instead, they rallied support. They pulled together the efforts of my co-workers, friends and family. The entire community chipped in. They collected enough money to cover my HBOT costs for two months.

The First Treatment

Of course I don't remember that first treatment. My mother rode with me in the ambulance from the hospital to the treatment facility. I imagine she was filled with both overwhelming hope and anxiety. There are no guarantees with HBOT.

My mother sat inside the chamber with me. She filled a sponge with water and placed it in my mouth while I was in there. The chamber resembles a little pod. There's a window so doctors and family can see inside. The water made me swallow, which equalized the pressure in my ears during the treatment.

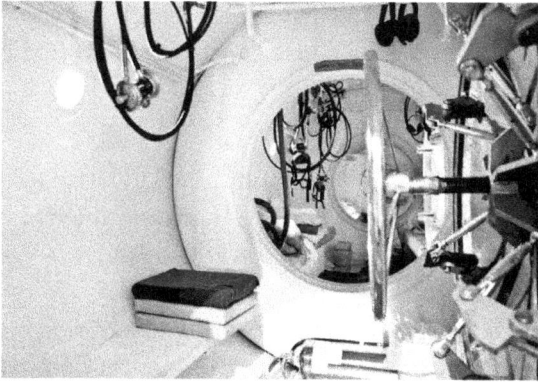
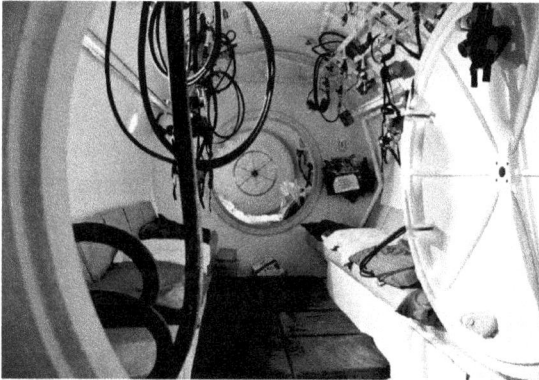

Inside the hyperbaric chamber

While I'm sure no one truly expected me to come out of my coma after the first treatment, they had to have felt some disappointment when I didn't. It must have been difficult to not see any improvement.

The Second Treatment

The second day, it was the same procedure. My mother rode with me to the treatment facility in the ambulance. She used a sponge to help me equalize the pressure in my ears.

Again, there was no real improvement. I was still in a coma. Patience is a virtue and it's always most difficult to find when your loved ones are at risk. Yet patience is exactly what was required. I'm not sure if I could have been as patient as my family is and was.

The Third Treatment

On October 30th, 2006, I awoke. See, I told you I was impatient! My eyes had been tracking to the left prior to the treatments. After the third treatment, they began tracking to the right and left. They began to focus. To doctors, this is a sure sign of improved brain function. After just three treatments, I came out of my coma.

After that, the progress was both significant and gradual at the same time. At first, I could only move the thumb on my right hand. After the eighth treatment, I was able to move my toes and my right leg. This was pretty significant progress considering where I'd been just a week prior. Still, there was a long way to go. I was on a feeding tube. I couldn't speak and I couldn't walk. Communication was difficult, but where there's a will there's a way, and no one has ever accused me of not having any will! (Quite the opposite actually.)

The treatments continued. Five days a week for two months, my mother traveled with me via ambulance to the HBOT treatment center where I would receive treatment. My brain would receive the oxygen it needed to repair itself. I'd return to the hospital.

After eight weeks of treatment, I took a six-week break. It was at that point I started looking forward.

Wheels In Motion

I've always been a fan of Rick Hansen. Rick is a Canadian Para-Olympian. He suffered a spinal cord injury in a car crash when he was fifteen that paralyzed him from the waist down. He was motivated to start a foundation, the Rick Hansen Foundation and the Man In Motion World Tour. He was also one of the torchbearers and brought the flame into the stadium to light one of the final torch lighters in the 2010 Winter Olympics

He's an amazing man to say the least. He inspired me, from my wheelchair, to make a difference too.

SPRING 2007: Just three months after awakening from my deep sleep, I decided to assemble a team for The Rick Hansen "Wheels in Motion" event held in Vancouver every year. My main goal was to improve the quality of lives of those with by spinal cord injuries, as that organization also does research to help these people.

The first thing that I did, which was quite successful, was to appoint my father as "PR" manager. He helped me to develop a winning strategy without putting all our cards up front. We kept a few in our back pocket, which we showed at the last minute.

The next thing that I did was to appoint someone on my team from within every major city in Canada and have some representation there, whether it was a family member, a friend, or a co-worker.

We collected donations for Rick's organization on a daily and weekly basis. These funds were deposited weekly into the bank and tracked by the foundation on a weekly basis.

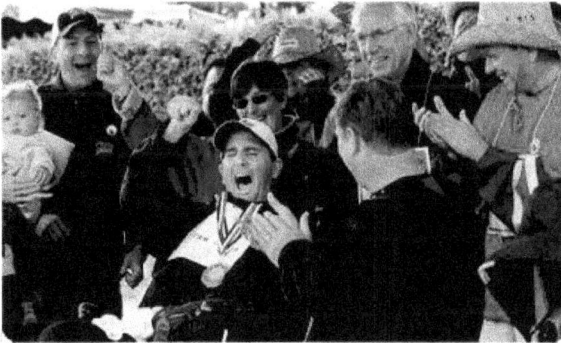

We then entered a team into a wheelchair race, which was held at the Pacific National Exhibition grounds in Vancouver. This picture above is from the event.

When the final tallies came in, the team that I had assembled from my wheelchair had raised just over $22,000.00.

Not bad for someone whose parents were told to put him in a long term care home for the rest of his days and who were told that he would never be able to contribute to society.

But my experience with TRHF gave me the idea and the insight to start my own Foundation (see www.secondchancestepbystep.org).

Rick continues to be a hero and an inspiration to me, and he also gives me drive and determination like my children do, to keep working hard at my rehab everyday so I can return to a more normal way of life.

I would like to thank all who contributed financially to Rick's organization and who devoted some time and energy to "Team Cosco's" cause and winning strategy.

When I look back, I think I was motivated by the fact that I was so grateful for getting my life back. I wanted to do something to make a difference. I also wanted to have a purpose, something to drive me. As you may have noticed, I'm competitive and I don't sit still easily.

This was the perfect opportunity to get really motivated and excited about something. It's easy to let negative thoughts and emotions take over. It's easy to look at your present circumstances and feel down and out.

It's easy to feel helpless.

But that's not who I am. I've never bought into the self-doubt, pity and helplessness. It just doesn't occur to me.

Wheels in Motion was the perfect opportunity. And boy did we blow them out of the water! When the event was over, we were the top fundraising team in their entire history. It was a very rewarding experience and it gave me the idea and insight to start my own charitable foundation.

But the work, both for the foundation and for my recovery, was just beginning.

~**Personal Essays**~

I first met Michael when I was undergoing Hyperbaric Oxygen Therapy for a neck and brain injury. At our first meeting, he was on a gurney and could only move his eyes. I spoke to his parents and found out the history of his circumstance.

I saw him twice a week for six weeks and I always said hello and goodbye to him. Over the six weeks, I saw his gradual improvement. I witnessed his sense of humour when he called one of the therapists at the Hyperbaric Oxygen facility "The Torture Lady."

I witnessed a lot of courage on Michael's part, as well as his loving parents Bob and Suzie. This experience has always stayed in my mind. Imagine my surprise and joy when I met Michael for the second time in the Stand Up for Mental Health Comedy course that we were both taking.

We both recognized each other and Michael, being the gregarious fellow that he is, immediately engaged me in conversation to figure out where we had met before. I felt that I was witness to a miracle when I saw him in his wheelchair being mobile and able to talk.

I thoroughly enjoyed being a classmate of Michael's for the year that we took the Stand Up for Mental Health class. I feel privileged and blessed to know him and his parents. Their positive outlook and courage in a situation that seemed hopeless has helped me to cope with my daily struggles.

To me, the word that best describes Michael is "courage." From the first meeting I was impressed by his courage to face and to eventually overcome a potentially devastating situation.

God Bless you Michael. I'm so glad that I know you.

Love,
Filomena Black

I remember the first time that I saw Michael a couple of years ago. He came into the clinic on a stretcher and needed help from us and the ambulance attendants to get into the chamber. One of the attendants couldn't believe how much he had already improved from the last time he had the privilege of driving him (he was speaking both French and English).

I went into the chamber with Michael, and over time I got to hear his amazing story, and about his road to recovery. His parents Bob and Suzie were there every step of the way, and it was very obvious that he had a very strong and loving support system.

Day by day and month by month, the changes in Michael were incredible!! I have never met someone who has such a strong will, and just pushes himself. Oh, did I mention that he also has quite the sense of humor? He lights up the room each time he is around and he is such an inspiration, not only to us at the clinic, but also to everyone who's lucky enough to meet him.

We are now in 2010 and just like Michael said, "he will walk out of this clinic," so it didn't surprise me that he has. He barely needs any help to get into the chamber, and his improvements on every level are just amazing to see.

He's so strong, and has worked so hard that it's wonderful to see all that hard work pay off. He has definitely shown me to never listen to what limitations someone else puts on you, believe in yourself and you will BEAT ALL ODDS!

Way to go Michael! I'm so proud of you, your success, and everything else you will accomplish.

Your friend,
Kelly

I met Michael Coss in the spring of 2009 when he came into our Hyperbaric Oxygen clinic with his parents, Susie and Bob. Michael literally lit up the room with his spectacular energy and gave everyone a 'thumb's up!'

Michael continues to be a most powerful energy and inspiration in our clinic to everyone he comes into contact with. Michael continues to teach without teaching, as his enormous heart touch the hearts of all who meet him. Michael's courage is also an enormous source of inspiration for so many as he continues to have faith in his healing journey.

Michael's laughter is a constant reminder to live life on life's terms, and that whatever those terms are, to live your best life, one step at a time.

We have a photo of Michael with 'his story' in our clinic, and so even when Michael is not in the clinic himself, he still continues to inspire people to take one step at a time on their own healing journey's finding themselves way beyond their original healing expectations. And it all started with Michael's determination, faith, love and courage!

Michael, knowing you has changed me for the better and I feel blessed to have had our paths crossed. I look forward to continuing to witness your journey as you beat every odd that has been put in front of you. You ROCK mon ami!!

GO MICHAEL GO!!

Lorraine Mock
Clinic Manager; Life Coach
www.hyperbaricexperts.com

CHAPTER FIVE

Finding My Way Back

*"Great changes may not happen right away,
but with effort even the difficult
may become easy."*
-Bill Blackman

When I woke from my coma I was able to move the thumb on my right hand. That's it. I had to re-learn everything. It's been a long haul. I've had more than 270 HBOT treatments and worked with more therapists and medical care givers than I can count.

I'm still not out of the woods yet. I still have goals and a long way to go.

There are so many therapies that have helped me over the past few years.

In the Beginning...

When I awoke, after those first few months of treatments, everything had to be relearned. Everything!

I was a preferred client for Band-Aids, as I had several cuts over my face and neck as I re-learned how to shave. I also had to re-learn how to dress myself and make myself look presentable. I re-learned how to use a toilet and washroom, but in the very early stages I urinated into a bottle in bed. Thank goodness I was able to master that skill again!

After my six-week break, I began HBOT again. Within six months I started physiotherapy. Physio is also called Physical Therapy. It includes physical therapy exercise, massage, and other modalities.

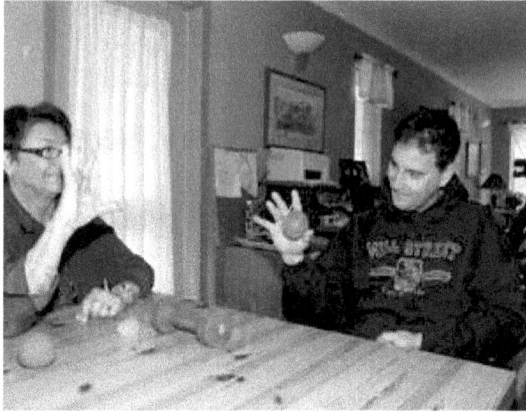

I also started occupational therapy. Occupational therapy teaches (or re-teaches) people to manage basic tasks. They include, but aren't limited to, work tasks, leisure tasks, self-care, and so on. For example, learning to shave is an occupational therapy task.

And yes, they keep you busy when you're recovering from TBI! I started speech therapy, too. By March 2007, I was able to finally get rid of that feeding tube and eat pureed food instead. Though I have to tell you that the first word I managed to speak several months later was not "applesauce." No I wanted a steak and I told them so.

In 2008, I started using a trainer to walk. By 2009 I was riding horses as part of my therapy. 2010 has brought a lot of advancements. I'm now using some amazing technologies and am making great progress. I will walk unaided again.

You may even see me at the finish line of the Boston Marathon soon! Don't be surprised!

What a Wonderful World It Is

Technology is a grand thing, especially when it helps people regain their lives. There are a few things I want to discuss because they've made a tremendous difference in my life. Because this book is about hope and inspiration, I felt it important to share these therapies with you. If you or someone you love is a TBI survivor or has had a spinal cord injury, they can make a world of difference.

The Watsu Pool

Presently I attend Watsu pool therapy once a week. Watsu is a gentle form of body therapy performed in warm water (around 35°C or 94°F). It helps relax muscles, which is good for spasticity. It combines elements of massage, joint mobilization, shiatsu, muscle stretching, and dance. You're supported while being floated, cradled, rocked and stretched.

The warm water helps to release muscles and joints. It reduces stress in both the mind and the body and is a part of physiotherapy programs around the world. It helps relieve pain and improves strength and flexibility.

When I'm in the pool, I can actually walk. It's like you gain supernatural powers within the water. I get a lot of satisfaction and gain my confidence back from being on my own two feet again. I also go to a city swimming pool once a week with a family member, as we find water to be an excellent medium in which I can re-learn how to walk. I remain very optimistic and confident that I will one day walk with my children to the park.

Speech Therapy

I am getting advanced speech therapy once a week, and I find that very beneficial. I look forward to the day that I pick up the microphone and liven up the room. Being a sales representative at

Molson, I further developed that confidence and skill. When I was much younger, I despised being the center of attention and would turn several shades of red very often. But now as I grow older, I am quite confident and enjoy being the center of attention.

When I first met my therapist, Dan Carlson, it was only a few months after my accident. Communication was seriously limited. We had a system of a thumbs up for yes and nothing for no, but it didn't always work. I started working with Dan about three times a month and we worked out a new communication system.

Around this time, I was getting REALLY tired of pureed food. So when Dan asked me what my first real meal was going to be, I spelled "steak" and then broke down crying.

This was a turning point because my family was finally able to tell that the old "Michael" was still inside a rather limited body.

Once again, doctors underestimated me. Progress with my speech therapy was slow and they began to assume that my ability to speak would be severely impaired. They figured that because it was already seven months out from the accident that any progress I'd made to this point would be all I could accomplish.

They were wrong!

On Christmas Eve in 2007, while Dan was away, I said my first word. I began speaking. It was a wonderful present for everyone. Speech still isn't my strong point and I'm still practicing. In fact, I practice alone in my room at night. I'm sure some of the sounds coming from my room sound quite crazy, but I'm determined to improve. I want to give speeches and talk about my experiences, so I have a lot of motivation.

The Lokomat Machine

The Lokomat is a walking treadmill. It's a therapy that I also take once a week. It's also called robot-assisted walking therapy.

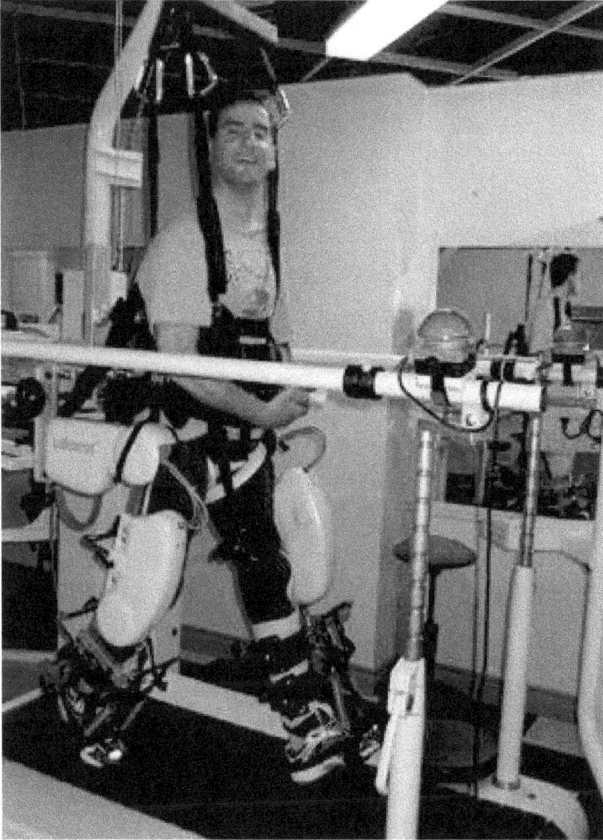

It's a form of physical therapy that works by essentially being strapped into a harness. Your legs and arms are strapped to the machine. It then simulates natural walking movements.

A computer controls the pace and measures my responses to the movements. It's believed that the repetitive walking pattern helps the brain and spinal cord work together to re-route signals that were disrupted by TBI and other injuries.

You can see a great video of me on the Lokomat machine on my Facebook page, The Courage to Come Back (Michael Coss). I invite you to stop by and check it out. It's also a great way to get involved in my foundation.

Kinesiology

In addition to helping forge new connections in the brain, this therapy helps strengthen muscles, bones and improve circulation.

In September, I started with Applied Kinesiology. Kinesiology is essentially the study of human movement. It essentially measures my movements and provides feedback. The kinesiologist I work with, Denise, is great. She taps into mind-body techniques to help clear emotions that are blocking success. She's also been working with me to improve my range of motion.

This therapy has worked together as an integrated approach with my neuro chiropractor and naturopath, whom I saw once or twice a month or as the need arose. The naturopath put me on some supplements to also help my recovery.

I strongly believe this is going to take my rehab to another level. When I walk several times a day, to and from the kitchen, to and from the washroom, and to and from my bedroom, fingers in my left hand would get so tense that my finger nails would dig into my hand. The pain from me re-learning how to walk would override any gains that I had made and would cause me major discomfort. With their help, this is beginning to disappear.

Right now my days are full of Lokomat, Watsu pool, speech therapy, and horseback riding. In addition, with visiting with my friends and family, writing this book, and building my foundation, I have very full days and a very full life.

I want so badly to learn to walk again. I want to take my kids to the park, and push them on the swing sets, to play softball, tennis, ice hockey, and play touch football with my friends and co-workers.

I am gaining more confidence standing and taking a few steps, and being in an upright position.

My rehab is going very well. Although I get frustrated at times, I have come a long way. From being in a coma, I am now eating and speaking. Doctors are baffled and do not know what to say. I am getting great therapy and I am always looking for other avenues that are going to take me to the next level. My long-term goal will be to travel to Kamloops and go see Dr. Chevalier, the neurosurgeon at Royal Inland Hospital. He was the first doctor to fight for me and was very good to my family. It'll be great to walk into his office and see him. He will think he's seen a ghost.

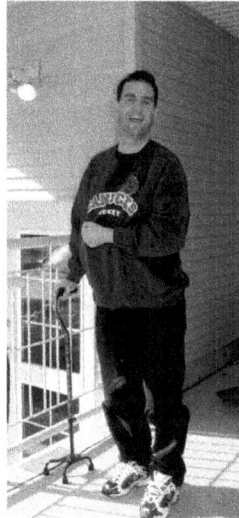

I am now walking with a single cane, instead of a quad cane, several times a week up and down the hallway—boy does that take effort, focus and concentration—but at least I'm taking steps. Actually, as of December 2010, I am making real progress toward my goal of walking.

Today is Friday, December 10th, 2010, and it is a very big day for me. After being in my comfort zone ever since my injury, I have decided to take the next step, which is to walk as much as I can, to the kitchen, to the bathroom, to my bedroom, and also to the living room.

I feel very confident with my decision, as my sense of balance has greatly improved. I also would like to add that I walked today with no cane or assistance. Boy, what a great feeling!!

I feel very optimistic with all my progress that one day I will walk with my children to the park hand in hand.

My confidence is increasing with every step that I take, inch by inch and day by day. This is probably the biggest and best decision that I have undertaken during my rehab, but I also realize that it will benefit me and my relearning of my walking ability.

Before I share a few essays written by various therapists, I would like to THANK Pauline Martin and all her staff at The Neuromotion facility, who worked with me in re-learning how to walk and all my Physios who have worked with me over the last three years. They've worked hard to help me put my body back into game shape. They're helping me relearn how to do the simplest tasks, as well as the most difficult ones. I am not quite ready right now, but I assure all of you that I will be ready and able to one day.

~**Personal Essays**~

My name is Mary-Lynn Corpuz.

I am a Rehabilitation Care Worker. I work for one of Cheshire Homes Society group homes called Larkin House, which is a home for people with traumatic brain injuries. It was 2007 February when I was assigned to work with a thirty eight-year-young man with a TBI after being in a MVA.

I was told he was severely disabled and that he had come out of a six-month coma, and was able to communicate but minimally. I was excited to meet this young man, but saddened to hear that the medical profession said that he would remain in his present condition with little or no progress. They obviously did not know Mr. Michael Coss.

When I met Michael, there was a twinkle in his eyes that shone to his soul and told me this was not an ordinary young man. I could see beyond his disabled body, a left side with contractions and very little movement, a right side also contracted, and a right leg that would constantly be kicking out.

His sense of humour came through within the first week of his stay with us when I told him that his right leg could kick his own behind to get him moving.

He started to laugh and couldn't stop, and that broke the proverbial ice. He has not stopped the mirth since and realized that all humility was balled up and thrown out the window as he took on the challenge of his life. Almost every day, there was some mark of progress that has defied his diagnosis. I could go on and on about his hurtles and his stumbles, but he can best tell it in his own words.

What I have to say about Mike (which I can now call him) is that I have been blessed with, not only working with such a

Continued

wonderful human being, but I am honoured to say, he has become a good friend and someone who has inspired me on many levels. I know he will always be reaching to meet the next challenge and will give everything is has to aspire to be the best he can.

Thank you, Mike. You have taught me so much and I will always have you in my heart.

My name is Denise Cambiotti.

I am a Specialized Kinesiologist. The way I practice this modality means I blend a "western" approach about body knowledge—most specifically about anatomy and physiology—with an "eastern" approach about body knowledge, which includes understanding the acupuncture meridian system and the chakra energy system.

I was invited to be part of Michael's team more than two years after his accident. Together with a naturopathic doctor and a chiropractor, who are both extremely experienced and leaders in their fields, we started working collaboratively with Michael in the autumn of 2008.

Michael has always been alert and inquisitive about his treatments with me, and displays tremendous commitment. Even before he knew what was in store during this step of his rehabilitation, he was willing to do whatever was asked. He is very motivated, and regularly requests work that he can continue between weekly treatments.

The particular reason I was invited to work with Michael is because of my training in advanced energy-kinesiology approaches, specifically "L.E.A.P. Brain Integration" created by Dr. Charles Krebs, who USED to be a quadriplegic himself. This modality enables a skilled practitioner to evaluate many neurological pathways, and then using "Applied Physiology" techniques developed by Richard Utt L. Ac., to defuse the stress that is discovered.

The effect is to encourage neurological signals to work more effectively. These two leaders in the field of Specialized Kinesiology (Utt and Krebs) have done a great deal to legitimize

Continued

the process of 'muscle-testing.' They've conducted enormous amounts of research and have created professional techniques that can be competently performed by just about anyone desiring to do this type of work.

A requirement to do this work competently is attendance at a few thousand hours of workshops, a desire to work as accurately as possible, a measure of common sense, practice, as well as a sense of heart! In Canada, practitioners of these modalities, as well as other modalities ranging from introductory to area-specific can be found at: www.canask.org

An important aspect of the work Michael and I have done together has been to clear emotional stress that has been bottled up in various body areas. This emotional work is non-invasive, but surprisingly 'deep.' Michael is never afraid to face and clear these emotional blocks. He will be the first to tell you how impressively his range of motion increases whenever we spend time working on clearing un-useful emotions!

One of the main words I could use to describe Michael is: "inspiring." There are many other words I could use to paint a picture of this young man who continually reveals interesting aspects of himself during his sessions. It is truly an honor to work with Michael as he regains control of the left side of his body.

Michael will not remember our first meeting.

He was in a coma. I was working at Royal Columbian Hospital and treated Mike during my weekend rotation. I would come up to the sixth floor and give chest physiotherapy to prevent him from getting pneumonia while he was attached to a tracheal tube. Sometimes I performed range of motion exercises on his arms and legs, or helped adjust the splints he wore to help prevent his muscles and joints from tightening up. Sometimes I got out the wheelchair that the nurses used for Michael to sit in, to help change his positioning and decrease the abnormal muscle tone.

Some months later, I was asked to come and work with Michael at Larkin House. I officially "met" him for the first time. Michael was sitting in his wheelchair, talking, joking, laughing, and very determined to participate with his recovery. This was the man I was going to work with over the next few months. What a change already!

I started coming to Larkin House twice a week for Mike's one hour physiotherapy sessions. We initially used a mechanical lift to carry him from the chair to the rehab bed, and practised sitting balance as he could not sit up by himself. He performed exercise after exercise, repetition after repetition, to improve his core, range of motion, and motor function.

Pretty soon, I had to be creative to keep things new and interesting, using bands, balls, and weights for exercises. Mike was also starting to practice "standing" on a tilt table. This was a machine that started off flat, onto which Michael was strapped at his chest, hips, and knees, and then the table was slowly straightened into a vertical position. One can imagine what it felt

Continued

like to be putting weight on the joints that had not had any weight on them in over a year.

Needless to say, Michael tolerated about three minutes the first couple of times. A lot of preparation for such a short time! However, this paid off.

Michael was soon able to sit up on the bed without any support. He could push himself up from a lying position, and shuffle himself sideways, roll onto his back, and onto his side. We worked on getting him able to transfer from the chair to the bed, so that the lift was no longer required. Every new challenge was met with optimism and determination.

I have never heard Mike say "I can't do it." He was always willing to try, and every challenge was met with success. On the tilt table, Michael began tolerating longer and longer periods of time, stretching out his body, and loading up the bones and joints that we take for granted.

"Success!" he yelled. I think we had to repeat that stand about five more times to show everyone at Larkin House that day.

The next step was for Mike to practice standing on his own without the tilt table. It took two of us standing on either side of him. He brought his center of gravity slowly over his toes and stood up from the low bed! He got so excited that he let go, dropped right back onto the bed, and pumped his arm in the air.

From then on, the rehab session involved "standing practice," with one person, two people, or using the wheel chair for support. Michael practiced endlessly, never complaining.

Our time came to an end when I had to go on maternity leave. However, Mike continued on with his physiotherapy, working up to three or four sessions per week, going to the hyperbaric chamber daily, and many other therapy sessions as well. I learned a very important lesson from Michael. Never rest until you have reached your goal.

Continued

Then you just create a new one. For whatever the future holds, Michael has hope and determination on his side.

By Anne Wong, Physiotherapist

Michael arrived in one of our community based group homes in Feb 2007. He was just emerging from a coma. He was unaware of his surroundings. He required total care support and had extensive contractures of all his limbs. He was not expected to recover beyond his present condition, to be independent, or to walk again. Michael went through various stages of recovery from awakening to the vital person he is today.

His rehabilitation program has been comprehensive, providing a wide array of services from a multidisciplinary team which include physical therapy. The physical therapy program has been designed to identify problem areas and to develop strategies for Michael that would produce positive results, such as a new way to walk or to be mobile.

Michael is a fighter and he has worked diligently on his physical rehabilitation every day, which has included strengthening, stretching, balance and gait training, bed mobility, transfer training, coordination. As a result, he is regaining physical strength and endurance and is, much to the surprise of most professionals, walking today. The process has been slow but progress is steady and he is deserving of recognition for the demanding and tedious work he has done to get where he is today. He has accomplished his goal of walking again and just needs to continue to practice his new skill to make walking more habitual.

Physical Rehabilitation is hard work and the rewards are slow and difficult to see. However, Michael is making the most out of life after his brain injury. He gets up every day in a positive frame of mind and dedicates his day to his rehabilitation. He does whatever it takes to hold on and to regain back his physical ability. He keeps positive and motivated and in believing that tomorrow will be better.

Continued

Michael uses a wheelchair which serves as a reminder that the injury occurred. He does not accept the fact that he will not walk again and is working hard every day on his physical therapy rehabilitation.

Michael is living testimony to how a successful man can be knocked down but not out, and how to overcome and succeed no matter what life throws his way. Michael is working on accepting the new person he has become, with a whole new outlook on life and knowing that he is a vital member of his community with much to offer.

I am so impressed with his courage, his attitude, his perseverance, and his positive outlook for each challenge he faces every day. I have been touched by his determination and motivation, his playful spirit, and his positive outlook on life. Michael's personal experience translates into lessons we can all learn from. Never lose hope, never give up, stay positive, and make positive change for yourself. I believe that Michael transcends the following message: change the changeable, accept the unchangeable and remove yourself from the unacceptable. One day, Michael wants to be a motivational speaker to share his experiences with others and to help other survivors. I believe he will accomplish this, and in doing so will definitely give back to his community.

From the first time you meet Michael, your life will be transformed in a positive way. His life is intertwined with hope, courage, and is an inspiration to other survivors. Mike has overcome some major obstacles since his car accident and has made a choice to make the best of some really tough situations. He does and will continue to make an impact on people's lives with his continued story.

Sue McCrimmon
Cheshire Homes Society of B.C. (2009)

**Michael Coss – my part in his miracle recovery
by Dan Carlson, Speech-Language Pathologist**

I first met Michael in early December 2006, when he was admitted to the convalescent ward of Eagle Ridge Hospital. He had been transferred from Royal Columbian Hospital where he had spent seven months, mostly in a coma, starting to recover from the traumatic brain injury he had sustained in a motor vehicle accident. On admission, Michael exhibited a non-verbal communication status. In other words, he had no speech at all. At that point, it was impossible to tell what combination of cognitive, language or motor-speech difficulty was causing this complete lack of speech. Michael opened his eyes, looked at people, and seemed generally aware of their presence, but overall appeared to be still in a semi-comatose state.

Communication abilities were near nil with the exception of somewhat unreliable movements of the thumb. His family and staff at the previous hospital had worked out a system whereby he would put his thumb up for "yes" and simply did nothing for "no." This system was a bit shaky to start as Michael seemed to be answering "yes" for everything. Later on, however, it became more reliable, and then eventually wasn't needed at all.

I saw Michael for therapy approximately three times weekly during the month of December. As noted above, we started with the yes/no response, and then moved to a letter board where Michael spelled words using his thumb response. This was done with the help of the therapist who scanned the rows and columns of letters.

Early on with this system, our biggest breakthrough and emotional moment came when I asked Michael, "What is going

Continued

to be your first meal once you get off the tube feed?" He was able to spell out the word "steak" using this method, and promptly broke into a flood of tears. It was at that point that his wife Ann and I really knew for sure that he was still in there.

This was great progress, however the miracle part was still to come. In recovery from brain injury, it is generally accepted that most improvement happens in the first few months, with slower recovery occurring after that time. When Michael first came to ERH, his physical and speech abilities were severely impaired; this combined with the fact that he was already seven months post-injury, led his health-care team to the conclusion that the prognosis for any further improvement was guarded.

Thus I thought that we would be looking towards equipping Michael with an augmentative communication device; using real speech seemed out of the question! How wrong I was...

Over Christmas I took a few days off and when I came back I met Ann in the corridor outside Michael's room. She explained joyfully that, guess what, Michael was now talking! I could hardly believe it, but found that of course it was true. His first attempts at speech were short, only single words and short phrases. His breath support was quite reduced and he was able to produce only word per breath.

Michael's voice was very weak, and he had to be reminded constantly to produce a voice that his listener could hear. His resonance was hyper nasal, meaning that too much air was coming through the nose, and his articulation was very slurred. The natural rhythm of his speech was quite disrupted due to all these factors.

Nevertheless, with a bit of effort both on Michael's part and on the part of his listener, he could be understood! A diagnosis of

Continued

dysarthria of speech was made, a disorder in which weakness and in coordination in the body's speech mechanism lead to disrupted processes of speech, including articulation, voice, resonance, breath support and the rhythmic flow of speech.

Michael continued to work at improving these deficits in therapy and was eventually discharged to Larkin House group home at the beginning of February 2007. I was asked by the house manager to continue seeing him at that location, which I did until his eventual discharge from my caseload several months later. Goals of therapy carried on essentially as noted above, that is improvement in the areas of breath support, precision of articulation, clarity of voice and stress and intonation of words and sentences.

Michael made excellent improvement during this time, and at the time of discharge, his speech, though still noticeably dysenteric, was functional in all situations—with the possible exception of when he was very excited!

I am very happy that my path crossed with Michael's during the course of my career in speech-language pathology. Not all SLP's can say that one of their clients has experienced a real miracle recovery, and I am pleased to have been a part of Michael's. I am proud to have been his therapist and will continue to be his friend.

My key word for Michael is: Miracle! Stay in touch!

Dan

CHAPTER SIX

Home Away From Home

"Every memorable act in the history of the world is a triumph of enthusiasm. Nothing great was ever achieved without it because it gives any challenge or any occupation, no matter how frightening or difficult, a new meaning. Without enthusiasm you are doomed to a life of mediocrity, but with it you can accomplish miracles."
-Og Mandino

Recovery from TBI can take a long time. For me, it's been an ongoing process, and I'm kept busy working toward my goals every day.

In February 6, 2007, I moved from Eagle Ridge Hospital into an assisted living facility called Larkin House. Larkin house is close to my family in Coquitlam. My wife and children feel quite comfortable here. The group home is run by Sue McKrimmon, and she runs a great ship!

My key worker is Mary-Lynn Corpus, and she pushes me very hard so I can one day return home to my family. The rest of the staff here is excellent as well and provides me with superior care. I'm quite fortunate to have found this wonderful place.

There are two sides to living away from home. The benefit is that I am surrounded 24/7 by supportive therapists and caregivers. I receive around–the-clock care.

The downside, of course, is that I'm not with my wife and children. However, I am blessed because I am able to see them several times a week.

I wanted to take a few pages in this book to call attention to this facility and others like it. One of the frustrations for TBI survivors is the desire to be treated with dignity and respect. It seems such a simple thing and yet not every survivor receives it. The Larkin House is part of the Cheshire Homes Society.

"The Cheshire Homes Society of British Columbia is a non-profit organization. Our mission is to assist individuals with acquired brain injuries to achieve their optimal level of independence. We believe that personal freedom, quality of life, respect and dignity are critical components in achieving this goal for each individual we serve." (Source: http://www.cheshirehomes.ca/)

Their vision is:
Acceptance, Empowerment, Independence, Opportunities

The Cheshire Homes Society of British Columbia will strive to:
- Continue to improve and enhance our existing services.
- Develop community-based partnerships that create opportunities for survivors.
- Develop a variety of community-based residential rehabilitation options for the brain injured throughout British Columbia.
- Deliver quality-based outcome focused programs to increasing numbers of survivors.

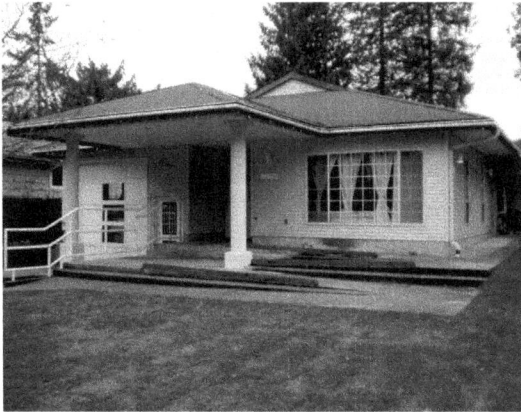

Larkin House—Michael's home for three years

Larkin House follows the basic guidelines below, and I can't tell you what a difference it's made in my life. To be able to live 'on my own' and have people around to assist me when I need it has been wonderful.

The Larkin House/Cheshire group of homes recognizes that each individual has:
- The right to be valued and treated with dignity and respect
- The right to personal independence and choice
- The right to reach their own personal goals
- The right to equal opportunity of access to services
- The right to confidentiality and privacy

The principles by which Cheshire manages are:
- Trust, honesty and mutual respect are fundamental for people to work together effectively.
- All residents, tenants, board and staff members have valuable contributions to make to the organization

Teamwork and participation are essential and promote belonging, self-worth and commitment.

Larkin House takes clients with all types of brain injuries. Candidates must be diagnosed with an acquired brain injury and be nineteen or older. Individuals must be capable of partial transfers for all programs, with the exception of Larkin House, which is equipped with a lift system. In some cases, a personal care assistant, such as home care or additional one-to-one hours, may be required in addition to the program costs. Recent medical and psychological reports must be made available upon referral.

Their programs are backed up by their research centre, run jointly with University College London, which helps them share good practice and innovations in the area of disability and development.

This wheelchair-accessible home was established in 1991 in Port Coquitlam as a permanent living facility. It is a four-bedroom, single-level house close to Coquitlam centre, providing complex care for medically challenged adults who are recovering from a brain injury.

While the program offers long-term support for individuals with severe brain injuries, the focus is on health and leisure. The program is supported by various therapists who provide in-house support, and includes a registered nurse, occupational therapist, physiotherapist, dysphasia consultant, art therapist, recreation therapist and a registered dietary nutritionist. An on-call physician is available in the neighborhood and a speech-language pathologist is also available on a consulting basis.

The clients participate in a day program in which they access community resources. A recreation therapist oversees the recreation program and day program. In house, they participate in various cognitive and physical programs based on personal choice, such as learning to use communication devices, improving range of motion, reading and watching movies, participating in music therapy and oral taste stimulation programs, following current events, developing computer skills, having visits from friends and family, and gardening. In the community, the residents enjoy swimming weekly, attending art groups, karaoke, adapted sailing,

> walking in the neighborhood and parks, and various social outings.
>
> http://www.cheshirehomes.ca/qs/page/1512/0/-1

Larkin House has been a positive experience and a step forward. I'm able to visit with friends and family in a comfortable environment. I'm supported to succeed and treated with respect and dignity. Thank you, Larkin House.

I must say that I am very fortunate to have such a great social circle and a vast network of friends. Family and friends have always come first to me. They came to see me at Royal Columbian Hospital and continue to see me here at Larkin House. These are people like Rachel Dumas, whom I used to call on at Jimmy Mac's pub and the Artful Dodger pub. The people that I can say stuck by me through thick and thin are few and far between, but their weekly visits and friendship are greatly appreciated. This chapter is a "Thank You" to all those people who come to see me on a regular basis.

I also want to acknowledge my brother Dwayne, who came to see me here at Larkin House and helped me learn to walk again in the local swimming pool. I recently started wheelchair curling with Dwayne, and although I used to be very competitive, now I strictly do it for fun and enjoyment. Dwayne lives here in Port Coquitlam with his special wife, Chantelle.

I also want to thank my other brother, Brian from Baie Comeau, Quebec for maintaining contact with me via phone several times through the week. I very much look forward to his very regular phone calls to update me on his family and job situation.

My parents have been and continue to be an ongoing source of support and motivation. They pick up my children and they all come and see me once a day. That daily visit means a lot to me as I get some quality time with my parents and children.

I also want to acknowledge the friendship of Ken Endo. He played softball and floor hockey with me. I want to thank Ken and his spouse Linda for their continued friendship. You both exemplify special people and I truly value your friendship and regular visits. The friendship of Joe, Vanessa, Graeme, and Karen are also greatly valued.

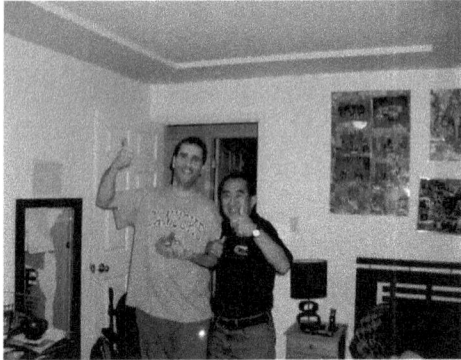

Michael and Ken Endo

I turned the big 4-0 a short time ago and I was able to celebrate my birthday with family and friends. We went to the Fraser Downs Racetrack and Casino for a group dinner, and a little gambling in the casino and at the horse track.

Seventy people showed up to my birthday celebration, which created some excitement and hype. My best friend Jay Heer (You might remember that I was going to visit him on the day of the accident) drove down from the city of Kelowna to be with me on my special night.

Still, I'm looking forward to the day I can once again live on my own and leave my room at Larkin House for someone else who needs it.

Discovering The Power in Me

While at Larkin House I've also undertaken two activities that I wanted to share with you. The first is a course I took called "Discovering The Power in Me."

It's put on by Worksafe BC. It was a two-day course that helps people facing the effects of long-term disability. It helps you find strength and resiliency within, so you can not only face your future with your head held high, but you can also set new goals and push boundaries you might not have otherwise established.

It really had a powerful effect on me. I can't believe the internal changes that happened over a two-day course. The course is set up to help you create positive life strategies, understand habits, attitudes, and limiting beliefs, and to increase self-motivation and confidence. I thought I possessed all these things in spades, but it really pushed me to have more. It lit a fire under me!

The course enabled me to break away from my comfort zone, my wheelchair, and I am now walking a minimum of three hours per day with a single cane. Boy, it's a powerful feeling being back on my own two feet again.

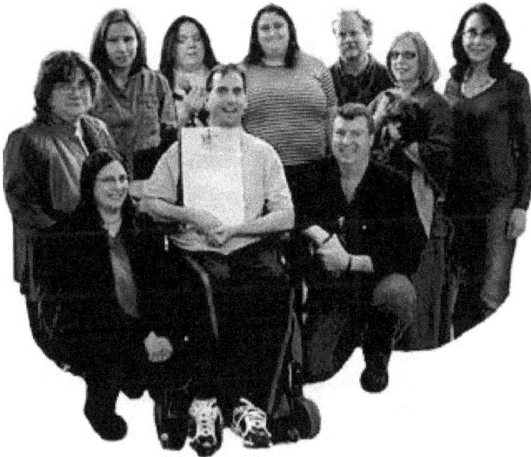

Stand Up For Mental Health

I also took part in the Stand up for Mental Health program.

Counselor and Stand-Up Comic David Granirer offers this program as a form of therapy. In David's Stand Up For Mental Health course, mental health consumers turn their problems into comedy, then perform their acts at conferences, treatment centers, psych wards, for various mental health organizations, corporations, government agencies, on college and university campuses, and most importantly, for the general public.

(http://www.standupformentalhealth.com/about.shtml)

"We use comedy to give consumers a powerful voice and help reduce the stigma and discrimination around mental illness," says Granirer. "The idea is that laughing at our setbacks raises us above them. It makes people go from despair to hope, and hope is crucial to anyone struggling with adversity. Studies prove that hopeful people are more resilient and also tend to live longer, healthier lives."

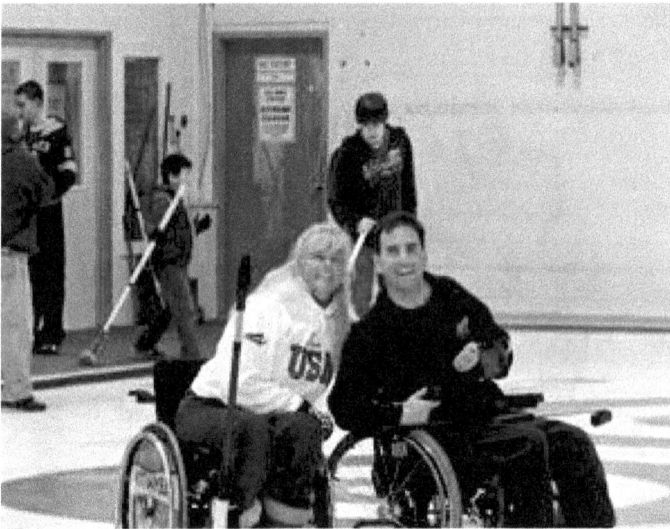

Wheelchair Curling

You know what curling is, right? It's that odd Canadian sport that makes the rest of the world scratch their head and go 'huh?'

But it's fun and it's competitive. You know how I love competition! Actually, I mainly do it for fun and to get out and be social. I've met some great friends along the way.

From Larkin House, where I lived for three years, I moved to The Connect brain injury facility in Langley, BC.

As you can see, I've created a good life for myself. I'm in therapy a lot, I have an abundance of opportunities to socialize and be with friends and family. I enjoy outings, sporting events, and am pushing my boundaries by taking courses and learning new ideas and concepts. All of these steps, both small and large, are helping me live a better life. They're helping me reach my goals of one day living with my family again, walking, and improving the lives of others along the way.

~**Personal Essays**~

How I met Michael Coss, October 6, 2008

My 2nd experience with wheelchair curling was when I traveled to Switzerland to officiate the 2008 World Wheelchair Championship in January. I witnessed the skills, courage, determination, excitement, challenges, and the laughter and camaraderie these athletes had developed. It was something that I will never forget. I had one player tell me he had never played sports, but after his injury someone had encouraged him to try curling.

He said, "It changed my life." It gave him a purpose. With lots of practice and encouragement, he made the USA Wheelchair team and won a Bronze medal in the 2008 championships.

As a life member of the Abbotsford Curling Club, I suggested we upgrade our washroom facilities and introduce the cub to wheelchair curling. In organizing our first league, we advertised for a "Have a Go Day." I got a call from Sue McCrimmon, manager of Larkin home in Port Coquitlam, and she had a person very interested in joining the league. Michael Coss.

She called several times with Michael's questions. Did I think he could do it? When could he come and try curling? Finally she put him on the phone. He was so excited to talk to me, but I was having trouble understanding him on the phone. When Michael gets excited his emotions take over and he communicates too fast. It was difficult to follow his conversation, especially being on the phone without seeing him. I was wondering if we could communicate.

He was in a group home for survivors of head injuries. Sue explained he could not use his left hand, but could attempt throwing a 40lb stone with his right hand. His brother would

Continued

bring him to Abbotsford. Dwayne and Michael arrived early just to talk and make sure they had time to talk before the start time. Michael is a real inspiration and joker.

Curling would challenge everyone who gave it a try. We started with easy skills, pushing the stone with a delivery stick. We then moved the distance to ¼ length, and asked the participants to try to push it to the rings from the shortened distance. It was hard, for many, but what was so rewarding for me was the look on their faces. The smiles and fun the athletes where having. The laughing, the kidding, and the competitive spirit of a competition. The enthusiasm they had to give curling a try. For many, it was the first time they had played a sport with family or friends. It was great.

Michael was quickly known as the fellow who could make the most fluke shots. He would come off a stone out of play and bounce to shot rock on a regular basis. We would all throw our hands up in jest and he would be telling us he called that shot. Laughing and proud to have made a shot.

The first day, he was not satisfied to throw to the shortened distance and wanted to see if he could throw the length of the ice. After a few tries, he made it and the satisfaction showed on his face.

I will never forget that first day of curling with this wheelchair group and their families. Curling is a game that can be played at many levels and Michael is why we want to bring it to a new level.

Michael contacted me when he began his foundation for a donation for his fund raising auction. I invited him to the farm to pick up my donation. He came with his parents and 2 children to see the cows and take a ride on my gator. Again he showed the strength he has to try something new.

Continued

He told me he is working hard for his for his family and friends. Yes, he is. You cannot turn back but move forward and be thankful for what you still have to change things you can but keep that positive outlook and you will succeed. I too always try to put things into the positive. You can always see things from the positive side if you look and try hard enough.

Keep it up Michael.

The word I use to describe you is "Positive"

He can do it!!!

Linda & Daryl Kirton

I first had the honour of meeting Mike Coss when we were both participating in the 2009 class Stand Up for Mental Health. His enthusiasm to simply be present and to socialize with others was tangible from the start. Soon, his ability to enjoy himself and to seek the humour in situations became more obvious as we went along.

At first, I was wrapped up in healing from my own dilemmas and somewhat protective about meeting people in a mental health group. Through time, however, I was able to meet some great people. Mike became one of my line-up mates, as his show-stopping comedy routine was usually immediately after mine. His routine curved back to more mainstream topics, after my comedy routine. My material involved sometimes uncomfortable-to-hear tales of recent ethnic discrimination in Canada and themes of sexuality. My husband once remarked, "Your routine may be one of the darkest in SMH, but Mike Coss' is the bluest of the bunch!"

As I got to know Mike, I thought about people in wheelchairs. Such as the challenges one faces when changing one's mobility from unassisted living and walking to a wheelchair. Mike, by the time I met him, seemed to be taking life's changes all in stride. On occasion, he would show emotion, but I did not sense a 'why me' or his feeling sorry for himself. I felt Mike was gracious and accepting of this phase of his life.

During creative writing sessions in SMH, Mike was only too happy to contribute to other student's material or to ask for assistance with his. Mike absolutely became one of the distinct individuals of the group. But moreover, we all were unique and distinctive individuals hailing from the different segments of Canadian society. Whether I met Mike before his accident or

Continued

after, to me he is a human being. I would have treated him the same either way—with kindness, sharp eye contact, and a snappy remark.

What stands out the most to me about Mike Coss is his ability to carry on—to carry on, no matter what. Many of us get caught up in the grief of our problems and traumas. We all certainly deserve mourning periods for loss and changes as they occur. Mike has the grace our present society embodies towards mobility impaired individuals on his side. Twenty to thirty years ago, the attitudes towards wheelchairs and the functionality for day-to-day living were not maintained or given precedence like they are today. If anything, positive people like Mike Coss who shrug off the difficulties life's challenges, help to further enlighten the masses.

My name is Eric Fielder.

I met Mike in early 2007 at Larkin House. I attended a team meeting with his therapists and family to assess his progress. Larkin House was then his home; it is a group residential home that houses the most severely disabled in our province. I was the vocational rehab consultant attached to Mike's case, representing WorkSafe BC.

I was told my job was to assess Mike's ability and prospects to integrate back to the community. Before I met Mike, his file led me to believe there was not much hope to expect—his injury and disability were so severe that he might well remain at a reduced mental and functional capacity forever. Indeed.

The meeting began and we sat around in a circle; Mike was in his wheelchair, his family next to him; we went around the room introducing ourselves. Each in turn gave his professional update— lots of medical, physical therapy, speech therapy updates, and cognitive assessments—they all noted his surprising progress. But when it came to predicting the future, what a sombre group we were, all business—except for Mike.

Before it was my turn to introduce myself, Mike's curiosity got the best of him. He looked at me and said, "What's your name? Do you have kids? After the meeting I'll show you a picture of my two, and my dog...Now, Eric, what do YOU do?" He knew my name! We all laughed.

I kept watching him through the meeting, his questions were direct as were his comebacks, and always his bright smile would light up the room, and when least expected, he cracked us all up with a double-meaning comment. He was witty. Seeing him laugh and cry, and how easily he expressed his emotions, made me think

Continued

this guy to be as compelling on stage as he would be in a room with a bunch of therapists.

Over time, we worked together on exploring what he would like to do and to where that might lead. Mike bought into the vision of becoming a stand-up comic, or has he says now, "a sit-down comic." Why not? He was a natural. They loved him in the class, once a week, where he arduously made the weekly trip to attend.

At the end of the year, he was acclaimed a star in the 2009 Stand-Up for Mental Health grad class, performing at least 10 venues in the city, with audiences of up to 200 people, and he continues as part of the alumni class. Now Mike continues breaking new ground, therapeutic horseback riding and soon, public speaking. You see, he has a story to tell.

Mike always speaks of an active life. He is active, pure and simple. Yes, in the past he was a pilot and adventurer. What is unique about Mike is that he pushes this self-image now and into the future—despite the odds, some real, but others only in the minds of the observer. For Mike, his active life is very much ahead of him, and is as tangible as the orange he will one day peel himself. I am convinced he will do big things. I am a convert.

5 little things Mike has taught me:

1) No matter what your situation, give back. Mike has fund-raised for Rick Hanson, reaching $22,000 in the midst of his own gruelling therapy and personal uphill battle. He inspires others with disability by just being himself, modeling. And he will inspire many more with his comedy and soon-to-be public speaking. He has independently been the lead point setting up his own Foundation to raise money for HBOT.

2) Be there for each other. Mike is a model on how to be

Continued

a friend. Also, he models how to offer support to those less fortunate. He arranges his all-too-infamous "pub nights" with his old friends, and makes many new ones in the process. Mike helps and encourages his housemates in countless ways and has shown he maintains lifelong friendships with those he worked for and works with.

3)   Don't stint with flattery. A genuine compliment can mean the world to someone. Mike knows this. He is not shy in acknowledging the support he receives and unabashedly thanks those around him for the support he receives, and each encouraging word. He looks at life that way; he is touched by those that go out of their way to make a difference and it will bring a tear to his eye.

4)   Rope others in. Mike will do what he can to engage any and everyone, bringing others into the fold of his friendship. He always has time for people, not only to support his own charity drives, but mostly, to just have fun with him.

5)   Always look on the bright side of life. As a person, Mike is engaging, welcoming, and fun loving. He is always looking up. And to boot, if the competition were held today, he'd win Father of the Year.

The word I would choose for Mike is MENSCH, a Yiddish word literally meaning Man, but stronger. "To be a Mensch" is to be a person embodying the characteristics one can look up to, to aspire to, and by his deeds, to offer an example to live by and learn from. Mike, you are a Mensch.

Eric Fielder

CHAPTER SEVEN

Letting Go

"You cannot turn back, but move forward and be thankful for what you still have to change things you can, but keep that positive outlook and you will succeed. I too always try to put things into the positive. You can always see things from the positive side if you look and try hard enough."
-Linda & Daryl Kirton

Many people who suffer from TBI struggle with depression. I'm lucky. While I have my moments, I've never really gone down that road. I guess it's not in my genetic makeup. It's not who my parents taught me to be. I've actually only had one really bad day.

For that I am grateful. It's difficult for many who are struggling with TBI to manage the day-to-day. It's difficult to look backwards at who you were before the accident and to then look at where you are now.

Things certainly change and change can be tough. To be honest...

I miss my job sometimes. I miss my co-workers and the interaction with them and my customers. It was a great job. I'm looking forward to being able to work again and all of the opportunities and decisions I'll be making.

I sometimes miss the relationship I used to have with my wife. Ann and I are going through the procedures for divorce and it'll likely be final around the time this book is published. However, we're the greatest of friends and will continue to be great parents together.

One common side effect of TBI is personality change. Sometimes it's a huge change; sometimes it's a minor change. I've changed. I love who I am. I'm really proud of who I am and what I've been able to accomplish. However, I'm not the same person I was when Ann and I married.

But I have something different now. Something that may be better. I'm able to make a difference in the lives of others with my foundation. I have a good relationship with Ann and my children.

There can be a lot of "if onlys".

There can be a lot of blame.

Recovering and managing TBI is about much more than physical challenges. So much can change in your life. Change brings a lot of emotional and mental challenges too.

Recovering and moving on is about letting go and holding on.

Letting Go

The inspiration, motivation, and purpose for this book are to give hope.

If you are struggling with TBI, it's truly important to let go of the "If onlys" and the blame. The past cannot be changed.

It's important to let go of the "Might have beens."

The "I used tos."

And the frustration.

Whether you believe in a higher purpose or calling or not, what you have and the only thing you will ever have is right now. This very moment.

Let go of the past. It's holding you back; it's holding you down. It's preventing you from seizing right now and making the most of your life. Trust me, there is still so much you can do and so many ways you can make a difference.

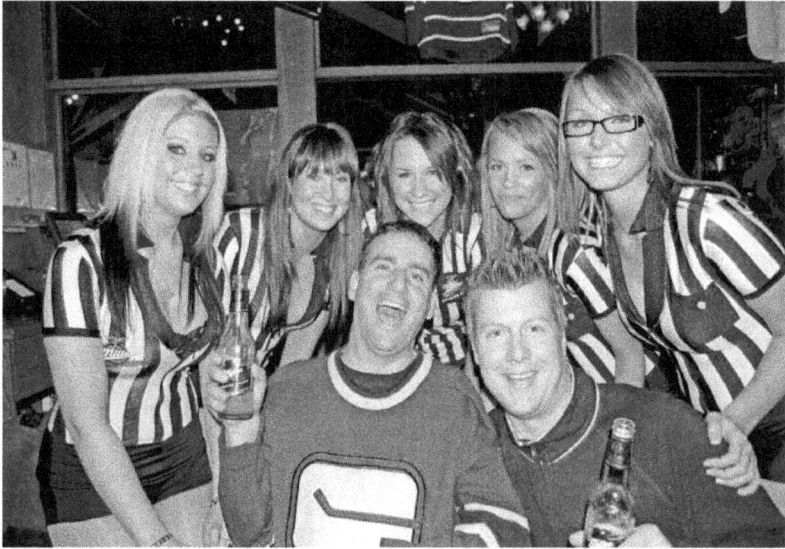

Holding On

And now here's the balancing act…

…the tightrope to try to walk.

Hold onto all that you are and all that you can be.

Hold onto your strength.

Hold onto your faith (in yourself and others).

Your loved ones.

Your caregivers.

Your motivation.

Your discipline.

Your positive outlook.

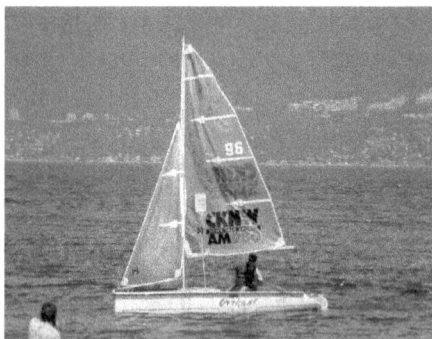

Hold onto the vision of a brighter future.

Hold onto your goals – both the big ones and the little ones.

The goal to walk one step forward and the goal to finish a marathon.

The goal to throw a ball or to play football with your friends.

The goal to write a letter and the goal to write a book.

The goal to say one word and the goal to eventually give a speech in front of thousands.

Hold onto the goal to make a new friend or to get married.

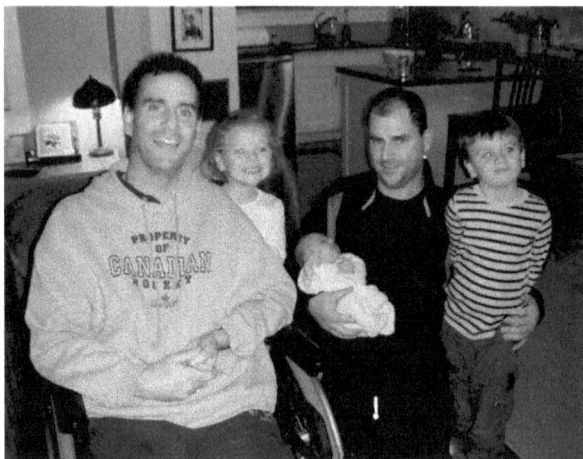

Whatever your goals are, hold onto them.

Hold onto your humanity. Release your humility.

Hold onto the courage and spirit you were born with.

Hold onto the person you are and the person you're destined to be. Things change. You choose how to respond to the change.

And if you find yourself struggling, if you feel your grip loosening, drop me a line. I'll be there to help you find your strength. I've been there.

Heartfelt Advice for Parents and Loved Ones of Those with TBI

My family is the reason why I work so hard on my rehab each day. My wife and children, my parents and brothers and their families, my friends and my co-workers are the reason that I get up each day and work so hard.

If there is some advice to share to help the loved ones of TBI survivors, no one is better qualified to share it than my mother, Suzette Coss. She offers the following sage advice:

> I would like to tell them to keep a positive attitude as it will help them focus on what they have to do to help their loved one.
>
> - To remember that doctors are not God, so therefore they do not know everything.
> - To talk to other families who have gone through the same thing. To be on the lookout for treatment outside our medical system. Go online and read testimonies of what other people have done, what helped.
> - To have faith and live for the moment.
> - To keep talking to their loved one, even if that person is in a coma. To keep massaging their toes, especially the big one as it sends signal to the brain.

- To have the professional show you the range of motion so that you can take over, because they are very busy.
- To be aware that his personality may change. Mood swings. Impulsivity.
- To take time for themselves, and for their relationships with each other, as a tragedy such as this will either bring you closer or break you.
- Remember it will be a long road. Rome wasn't built in one day. Don't be afraid to ask questions.
- One day you will meet the right person who will, in turn, put you in contact with someone else. Doors will slowly open one by one.
- Life doesn't end; it just takes you to a different path.

May God bless you,
Suzette Coss

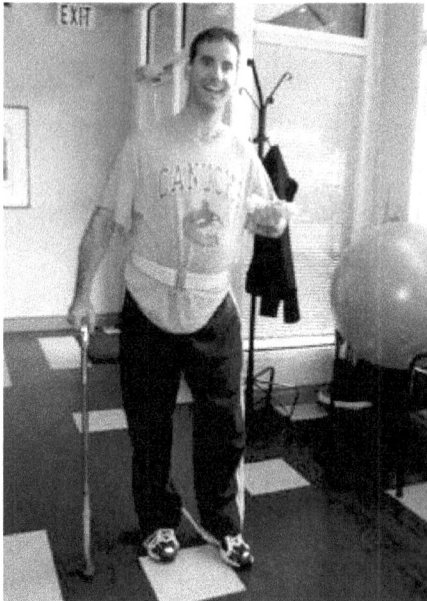

My Personal Advice to Those Struggling with TBI and Maintaining a Positive Mindset

My parents were told a few years ago by the medical experts that they should look for a long-term care home to take care of me for the rest of my days. They were also told that I would never be able to walk and that I would need help and some sort of assistance for the balance of my days on this earth. I am currently re-learning how to walk inch by inch, step by step, and day by day.

I am also currently re-learning how to swim—breath by breath, stroke by stroke, and kick by kick. Our brains continue to create new pathways to reach and activate those dormant neurons; therefore I have not stopped making progress. One day I will walk hand in hand with each of my children to the park.

Remain positive. Stay focused on your goals, and one day they will materialize, as there is light at the end of the tunnel. I've met some individuals who were once in a wheelchair like me, but have gotten out and who have re-learned how to do the most basic of things.

As for the doors that close behind you, like lost friends and contacts, new ones will open up to enrich your lives. I have met many people that I will learn things from and hence continue to grow and develop new friendships. I have lost many friends, contacts, connections, co-workers, etc., but the new people that have entered into my life are making a positive impact on me.

It may be a bit strange or odd to hear this, but I feel that I am a better human being as a result of my experience, a better person, and a good friend to the new people that I have met. And I will be a great father to my children, even if it means being in a wheelchair for the time being.

My children are the two people that motivate me the most, and I have a picture of each of them on my wall. They keep me focused, keep me grounded, with both feet planted on the ground. They put a smile on my face when I'm having a tough day, and those days are few since my injury.

It will not be easy by any means and nothing will be handed to you on a silver platter. You have to want to progress, and fight for every inch. I once accepted the fact that I will be in my wheelchair for the balance of my days, but **no more**. I am very confident that this is a temporary situation and that I will walk one day.

Set some small goals for yourself, and once you reach them, set some bigger ones, and give yourself a pat on the back once you achieve them. When I awoke from my coma, the only thing that I was able to do was to move the thumb on my right hand. Now I'm able to walk within water, and soon I'll be able to walk on land.

My advice to those struggling with a TBI and trying to maintain a positive mindset is to take things day by day, inch by inch, and step by step.

1. **Set small goals for yourself, achieve them, and then set some more goals for yourself.** Walk before you run. For example, I had to re-learn how to eat, and I looked like I was a poster boy for Gerber baby foods. I started out with a "puree" diet in which my food was put through a blender. This was so that my swallowing muscles would get used to eating again, as I had been stomach tube fed for quite some time. I couldn't imagine that going to a nice steakhouse for dinner one evening would have been a good idea.

2. **When you are having a tough day, which you will, think about something that brings you instant and immense joy and satisfaction.** For me, those are my children: my son Nathan, and my daughter Danielle. As I mentioned above, I have a picture of them on my wall, which makes me awaken each day with a smile on my face and starts my day off on the right foot. I envision myself walking up the front steps of our house hand in hand with each of my children and with our family dog not too far behind.

3. **Have an attitude of Gratitude**, be thankful of the people who are working with you each day. Don't be afraid to share how you appreciate the work that they do on a regular basis, whether you do so through your choice of words, a THANK YOU note, or a quick e-mail.

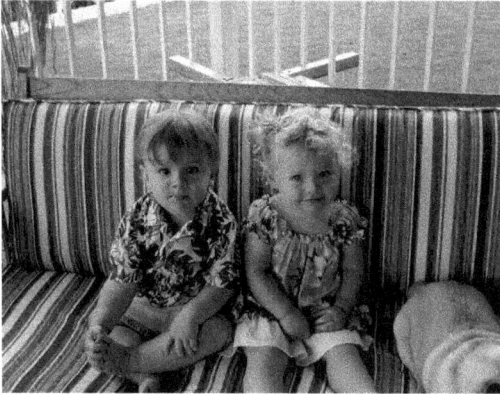

Nathan & Danielle

4. **Recognize your progress.** You and others will notice some improvements in your daily progress, which will be in many shapes and forms, which may be physical or even mental from a cognitive point of view.

5. **Never give up trying to improve yourself.** I often close the door to my bedroom and work on my speech. To others, it must sound like I am in a facility for those that have mental issues considering the sounds that are coming from my bedroom.
    Reward yourself with your positive gains, no matter how small they may be to you.

6. **Be happy with yourself, and the positive gains that you achieve and make.** I started out by weight bearing on a tilt table so that my legs would get used to me being in an upright position. And now I stand several times a day beside a wall, bearing all my weight on my own two feet.

And now I am re-learning how to walk, which doctors told my family members that I would never be able to achieve, that they should find a long-term care home to take care of me until the end of my days. And boy, if they saw me now, writing my own book, and walking on the Lokomat machine, or even horseback riding, or swimming...

My Inspiration

My inspiration comes from two people that I do not even know or have met.

Their names are Shannon Wiley and Karen Lennox. Shannon suffered a snowboarding accident a few years ago and it has taken her four and a half years to fully recover. Therefore I know that it can be done. She is back to work now as a paramedic with the BC Ambulance service.

Karen Lennox was in a motor vehicle accident in February of 2004. Her truck hit a patch of black ice. The trailer she was towing pushed her into oncoming lane, and she had a head-on with a loaded logging truck.

Both trucks were written off and hers was totaled. The logging truck had no steering after they hit, so it was a write-off too. Karen was driving a 2002 F150 at the time and it looked like it was melted all the way to the cab. Nobody knew she survived, but she did not have a mark on her, just a cut lip and a bruise on her forehead. She broke her C1, tore her brainstem, broke her pelvis, fractured 2 ribs, bruised her lung, tore the ligaments on one side of her neck, then she re-broke her ankle too, but that was minor anyhow.

She had motivation though. She was only in the hospital for just over two months. She was in ICU in Edmonton for three weeks, in the regular ward for a week, and then she was transferred to Glenrose for rehab and was there for five weeks. Then she went home. She was even kind of walking when they moved her out of

ICU: she had a physio on either side and that's how she walked.

The doctors told her they could not do anything for her, so she did it herself. It was hard sometimes, but then she reminded herself of where she wanted to be and then she pushed herself some more. Some days she had more energy than others, and some she didn't have much. But she kept positive and kept working at it, and it got better.

Shannon Wiley and Karen Lennox inspire me. Rick Hansen inspires me. But most of all, my family inspires me.

My biggest motivation also comes from myself. I must first do this for myself, find happiness, and then let it flow like a river.

Secondly, I must do it for my children, my son Nathan and my daughter Danielle so we can be together as a family. My children ignite the fire within me and keep the torch burning.

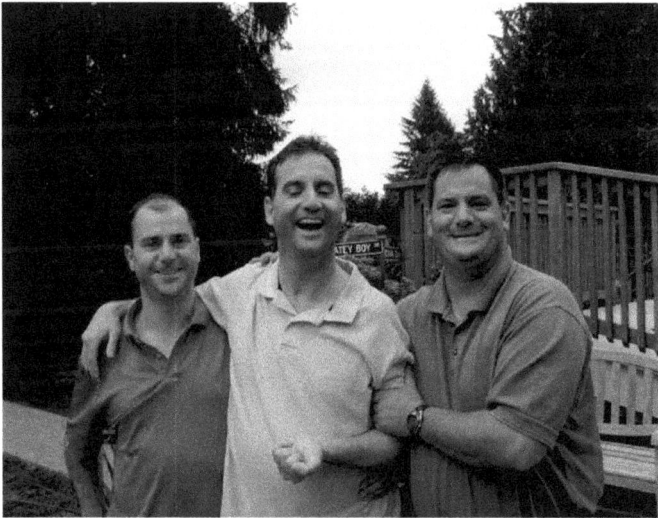

Michael, Dwayne & Brian 2009

CHAPTER EIGHT

For My Children

*"Cosco, It's been a while since I have seen you!
Always thinking about you! We keep on praying
for your recovery. Mike, you are looking good!
Keep on fighting, you can do it!"*
-Dan Derksen

Being a new father was a dream come true. I can say that it was a truly spectacular feeling. Ann and I had tried for several years to conceive. When we discovered she was having not one but two babies, we were overjoyed. We told anyone who would listen. It was a defining moment, to say the least. I'll remember that joy for the rest of my life.

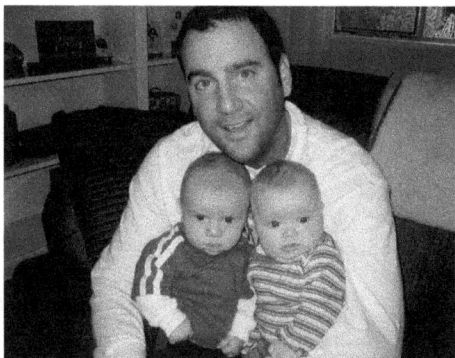

New parenthood brings with it joys, anxieties, happiness, and fears. It's almost overwhelming.

Yet at the same time, when you look at their little faces, everything in that moment is absolutely perfect. All is right with the world.

Both Danielle and Nathan are the lights of my life. They're the reason I get up every morning. They're the reason it's so very easy to laugh and smile.

I say that they're my motivation, however my motivation is really self-centered. I want to walk with them. I want to hold their hands and stroll through the park. It's an image I can see perfectly in my mind. The grass is green. The sky is a crisp robin's egg blue. Children are running through the park laughing and having a wonderful time.

Danielle, Nathan and I are walking together. I'm in the center between the two of them. They each have a hand and we're strolling and talking. We're headed for the swings, where I'm looking forward to pushing them until they go so high they squeal with delight.

They both have a twinkle in their eye and a smile on their face, because what child doesn't enjoy a sunny day in the park?

This vision, it's for me. It's what keeps me going. It's what has always kept me positive and motivated.

When I was in a coma a collage of photos hung on the wall. It was a collection of baby photos of both Danielle and Nathan. I'm certain having this on my wall helped to keep me going.

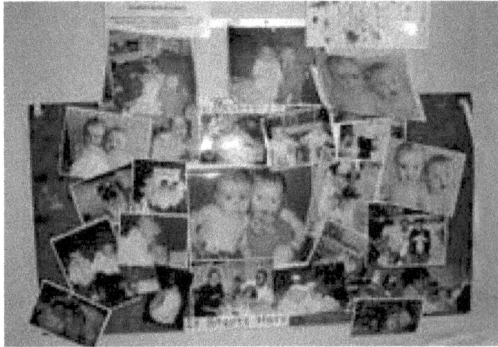

Parenting from a Wheelchair

I've been parenting my children as best I can from my wheelchair, as I am currently re-learning how to walk. The joy and excitement that I see in their faces as they climb over Daddy's lap while I am in my wheelchair makes my day and gives me the drive and determination to work even harder at my rehab, to try to learn new things to become independent again.

Ever since I woke up from my coma, I've been living in a group home that is exclusively for people who, like me, have experienced a traumatic or acquired brain injury. Some of the residents are exclusively stomach tube fed, non-vocal, and who will be in a wheelchair for the balance of their days.

I am in a wheelchair for now, but my goal one day is to walk and I remain very positive and optimistic that I will be passing on my wheelchair to someone that needs it more than I do. I go home one day a week (every Sunday) for around four hours, and I usually stay for dinner. My spouse comes to see me with my children several times a week, which solidifies the relationship that I have with the two of them.

I have their pictures on the wall of my bedroom, as they are the driving force as to why I wake up each day with a smile on my face and give each day 110% towards my rehab. They are my inspiration, my motivation, and why my rehab and my walking ability are so important to me. They are the ones that light the torch and fire within me.

As I've said, my future goals one day are to walk hand in hand with each of my children to the park and watch them swing on the swing sets as I stand behind them and push them. I also look very much forward to coaching them in the sports that they choose, just like my father was very much involved in the sports that I undertook. I also look very much forward to escorting my daughter down the aisle one day when she decides to get married to the person of her choice and being present and able to witness my son's wedding and graduation. I also will support them and encourage them in any play or band that they play in.

I will support and encourage the two of them in their profession or studies of choice. I will also support and encourage the two of them in their social circles and amongst their friends and relatives, as my relatives were very important to me while I grew up.

Watch Out Wayne Gretzky!

My desire to walk again, return home to my family, and return home to my work for Molson is the fuel that lights the fire within.

I work extremely hard every day to learn how to walk, and I feel extremely positive that it will be done. The weekly swimming pool sessions that I attend instill the confidence in me that it can and will be done. When you are weightless within the water, it enables you to do things that are non-existent or harder to do on land.

The work that I have been doing with Denise Cambiotti is starting to bear some fruit. I now have much more control over my left leg, which was barely non-existent before. Other people have noticed that my left leg has much more strength than it previously had. Some of the things that I see Denise doing—like tapping her heels together—I say to myself, "What does this have to do with my rehab?"

I recently found out that she is going to be working with Rick Hansen, and I am encouraged for those people who have been affected by a spinal cord injury. In my short time with her, I am starting to notice some positive changes and I realize that this is only the tip of the iceberg. She instills faith and confidence in me as part of her work, and I feel confident that she will move the needle more within me.

There is nothing more that I would like than re-learn how to walk, return home to my family, play with my kids, and teach my son how to ice skate and play hockey. I now look forward to lacing up my son's skates for the very first time and seeing him enjoy himself. Watch out Wayne Gretzky!!

Before sitting down to write this book, I asked many people to contribute. Their essays are distributed throughout the book. I'm so grateful for their contributions. They mean the world to me.

However, no contribution is more important than that of my parents, Bob and Suzette Coss. Because of them, I am here. Because of them, I am able to write this book and help others. Because of them, I am able to be a father to my two children.

I've asked my parents to share their story. Their perspective and the story they lived is quite different from my own. However, if you're a parent or family member of someone with TBI, then perhaps it can help you find the hope and inspiration you need to support your survivor.

As a parent, nothing in life prepares you for that phone call telling you that your child has been in a terrible car crash. You feel that it just cannot be happening to your family.

My husband and I got married very young and have three wonderful sons. We were living in the city of Quebec and were both working. I worked in a rehab center in the health records department. Bob is a customer service manager. You and Dwayne were both living in Coquitlam; B.C. Brian was living in Baie Comeau with his family.

On Thursday, May 18, 2006, Dwayne (our youngest son who was in Toronto on business) received the news that you had been in a terrible car accident. He phoned his dad, who came to tell me at work. News of the accident traveled fast, but information wasn't available to us fast enough.

You and your family were traveling to Kelowna with your seven-month-old twins. You worked as a marketing coordinator for Molson Canada, and were going to do a promotion and your wife and the twins were going to visit some friends. Catastrophe struck on the Coquihalla, and you lost control of the van, which rolled over at least one and half times.

Miraculously, Ann and daughter Danielle escaped with only minor injuries, but you and Nathan were not as fortunate. Nathan spent several weeks at BC children's hospital with head injuries.

When the medical services arrived at the scene of the accident, you were unresponsive, with evidence that the airbags had deployed and that you were restrained by his seatbelt. The Glasgow Coma Scale (GCS) rating at the scene was 8 out of a possible 15, indicating a comatose state. You were transported by air to the Royal Inland Hospital in Kamloops.

Bob and I were only able to get a flight for Vancouver the next day. We were in a daze. I don't recall the plane ride. I kept praying, hoping that this was just a nightmare or that someone had played a bad joke on us.

Upon arriving at the airport, we phoned the hospital and drove to Kamloops. You were in the intensive care unit. Dwayne and his wife Chantelle were already there. We had a tearful reunion and a nurse came to talk to us to explain our son's condition.

When we first saw you lying in that hospital bed, hooked up to all these different machines with tubes and needles attached to almost every part of your body, you looked as handsome as ever—not a scratch on your swollen face. You were unresponsive, but upon hearing our voices, your blood pressure went up.

We were told to be very quiet and not to touch you. But how can you tell a parent not to touch his child? I did, and I swear that you reacted by squeezing my hand very faintly.

The nurses and the hospital personnel were very kind to us and let us stay with you as much as possible. We had accommodations at the Coast Inn and Bob and I would stay with you during the day. Dwayne and Chantelle would spend the night.

It's very hard to focus on anything else; you act in automatic mode. You pray, eat, sleep, and keep hoping that it is just a nightmare.

On Saturday, we met Ronnie, Dave, and Heath from Molson and we found out about a side of you which we didn't know. They described you as a very generous, good and big-hearted human being always willing to help others.

They told us what a great guy you are, how many friends you have, that everyone loves and respect you, how dynamic, energetic and that nobody could beat your numbers. We were very touched.

We met Dr. Chevalier, a neurosurgeon from Quebec, who told us that you had a diffused brain injury. He said that your age, health, and physical condition would help you. You were stable but not responding.

We had to keep positive, because first of all you are a fighter, and secondly you have a wife and two children who need you. All we could do was tell you how much we love you, hope, and pray.

Before your discharge, we were told that it would be a very long road and that it would take a miracle. On May 30, you and I flew by air ambulance to the Royal Columbia Hospital in Vancouver on 6h north, which would be your home for the next seven months.

We moved in your basement suite. Jenifer also shared the suite with us. It was a very hard time for all of us. We were fortunate that dad was able to work in the office in Richmond. I spent my day in the hospital with you. I would talk to you about when you were growing up, the things we did as a family, and about your own family. I would rub your big toes.

I remember the first time Dad and I took you outside. They had a patio on the roof with plants. As we were waiting for the elevator, Ken came out and when you heard his voice you started crying.

You had a very good occupational therapist named Rebecca who got you the dyna splint for arm and your leg. She was very nice and always smiling.

You also had a physiotherapist named Anita. As the time went by, they taught me how to do your exercises and how to put on your splint.

At the end of October, Dr. Lee told us that there was not anything more the hospital could do for you and that they were looking at another facility for you to move to.

Dwayne's father-in-law happened to be watching a program on TV about hyperbaric oxygen therapy. He mentioned it to dad, who did a lot a researching about it. After spending hours and hours reading testimony, he was convinced that it was the route to go.

He called I don't know how many clinics across North America. He finally found one which agreed to send a doctor evaluate you to see if you would be a good candidate for this treatment. These treatments were very expensive and not covered by health insurance. Your friends from Molson had a big fundraiser for you. We had to sign release papers from the hospital, and finally it was arranged that you and I would travel by ambulance five days a week to get you the treatment.

When we first started going to the clinic at the end of October 2006, you were in a fetal position and your eyes were only tracking to the left. I would go in the chamber with you and put some water on a little stick with a sponge at the end and put it in your mouth so you could swallow and relieve the pressure in your ears.

After the third treatment, you started focusing. After eight treatments, you were able to move your toes and your right leg. We would go for forty treatments, take a six-week break, and start all over again. In December you moved to Eagle Ridge Hospital. With the help of a speech therapist, we started showing you cards with the letters of the alphabet on it. If it was the right letter, you would blink once for yes and twice for no.

It was a very slow and long process, and we added some cue cards with pictures on it. By Christmas Eve you were saying your first word. What a beautiful Christmas present.

You were having physio, occupational therapy, and speech therapy. You were being tube fed and you couldn't sit. In February, you moved to a group home in Coquitlam, and Sue the manager couldn't believe how you had progressed since she had come to the hospital to evaluate you.

Michael's motivation and competitive side finally awoke and kept on driving him. In the spring of 2007, Michael became involved in raising money for the Rick Hansen Wheels in Motion charity. With the help of his co-workers and friends, Michael became the Top Fundraiser in Canada and set a fundraiser record for the entire six-year history of the program. But his dad, who played the role of manager, did a terrific job in helping Michael get there.

Michael had to relearn everything and very slowly was introduced to pureed food. It was a long process, but eventually the feeding tube came out and Michael was finally able to enjoy his favorite food, steak on the barbeque.

Your younger brother takes you out and visits you regularly. Brian, who lives in Quebec, calls you about every two days. People move on with their lives, but you are lucky to have some very faithful friends who keep in touch with you— Rachel, Ken, Jo and Vanessa, Graham and Karen—may God bless them for the joy they bring into your life.

To this day, you have had about 270 hours of HBOT. Along with physio, occupational therapy, and speech therapy, we also tried kinesiology, acupuncture, naturopathy, Gi Gong, and neuro chiropractor. We just finished a treatment called neuro network.

They say to every adversity there is a seed of benefit. Well, this tragedy has brought us closer as a family and taught us to appreciate life STEP BY STEP, one day at a time.

Today you remember everything up until the accident and have gained a sense of determination that is unstoppable. You have to improve your short-term memory. You are hard at work on your rehabilitation program and can now walk, at your own pace with assistive devices and supervision, and your aim is to do it on your own, sooner rather than later.

You have one goal: to be healthy, regain your independence and WALK TO THE PARK WITH YOUR CHILDREN. You have taught us the meaning of the word RESILIENCE. You have strength, endurance, and perseverance.

You inspire and motivate others to tackle life's hurdles head-on and to never give up, always with a smile. And that's exactly what you've done, at least for all members of our family.

CHAPTER NINE

A New Purpose

"It's not whether you get knocked down, it's whether you get up."
-Vince Lombardi

Sometimes an amazing opportunity shows up when you least expect it. Sometimes, perhaps, things happen for a reason.

My accident changed my life. It's changed the lives of many others too. It's my goal, my purpose, and ultimately the silver lining to continue to have a positive effect on the lives of others. I've made it my mission to bring HBOT to people who need it.

HBOT gave me a second chance at life.

Doctors thought that my parents should look for a long-term care facility to take care of me for the rest of my life.

Fortunately for me, and for others, they didn't give up hope. They found HBOT and the rest is history.

Through that traumatic yet powerful experience, and my experience with The Rick Hansen Foundation, I was inspired to start a foundation.

I wanted to do something for brain injury survivors and promote and help fund HBOT, which is what my friends, family members and co-workers did for me. I realize that this type of treatment needs to be promoted, and also needs to be financially assisted, as it is not covered by Medicare and any private insurance.

My priorities remain:
#1 My rehab,
#2 My family,
#3 My foundation.

I feel that this type of treatment must be further explored and talked about. It should be tried by those families who have had a loved one affected by a traumatic or acquired brain injury.

The problem today is that Hyperbaric Oxygenation Therapy, though it is working, is not approved for brain injury, and as a result is not reimbursed by MSP and any private insurance. Because of the cost of such treatments, most of survivors that could benefit from them and regain a better quality of life cannot afford to pay for them.

Many of us still don't understand why doctors, hospitals, and the medical system as a whole don't acknowledge the proven benefits of HBOT, and refuse to give HBOT treatments to patients in the early stages following the brain injury.

In most cases, they will start physiotherapy and other therapies on the patients, which is a good thing without a doubt. However, without taking into consideration that the brain, which is the central system that sends signals to the rest of the body, need this priceless and powerful natural drug—oxygen—to be able to function.

Damages to the brain occurred in the first place because, at some point, it lacked oxygen for too long. It DOES NOT NEED MORE LACK OF OXYGEN NOW!

Oxygen is crucial to tissue repair. The brain is no exception to the rule. Pure oxygen given to a patient in a hyperbaric chamber, which increases the surrounding atmosphere's pressure, dissolves deeper within tissues and fluids. The oxygen can then help awaken dormant neurons in the penumbra area surrounding the direct damaged part of the brain and rebuild new connections. Over time, these new connections will take over for old ones that have been irreversibly damaged.

Although Hyperbaric Oxygenation Therapy (HBOT) won't increase the chances of recovery in some cases, in most cases HBOT should be attempted. Because it has been proven that, without a shadow of a doubt it works, it helps, HBOT SHOULD BE USED as soon as possible after a brain injury in CONJUNCTION WITH other rehabilitation treatments and therapies (Neuropsychology, occupational therapy, physiatry, physiotherapy, nursing, recreational therapy, social work, speech and language pathology, vocational counseling...etc). HBOT medical staff and brain injury rehabilitation teams should work together, hand in hand, for the benefit of the survivors and their families

For the vast majority, the first year is the crucial time for recovery. After one year, the window for improvement begins to close. However, in many cases, radical improvements have been noticed after HBOT treatments years after the brain injury occurred.

The Michael Coss Brain Injury Foundation

Do you have a CHILD with a recent or chronic BRAIN INJURY?

Within the scope of a clinic study on HBOT (Hyperbaric Oxygenation Therapy) applied to the brain following either TBI (Traumatic Brain Injury) or ABI (Acquired Brain injury), the *Michael Coss Brain Injury Foundation* is looking for children under 12 years of age who would qualify and benefit from this therapy.

ALL TREATMENT COSTS FOR THE THERAPY WILL BE PAID FOR.

For further information, please contact **Lorraine Mock** at **604-521-5177**

VISIT US AT
www.SecondChanceStepbyStep.org

Our Mission

To provide survivors of brain injuries help and support through the unique approach of Hyperbaric Oxygen Therapy (HBOT) in order to improve their quality of life and create a better future.

Our Vision

To reach out to those survivors of brain injuries who cannot afford HBOT, since it is not covered by our Medical System. HBOT allows the development of new blood vessels to the rim of tissue surrounding the area of the brain that has been damaged.

These newly formed blood vessels resulting from the hyperbaric oxygen therapy can then bring fresh blood (oxygen) and nutrients to the damaged tissue. The tissue begins to repair itself and returns to normal or near normal. These "resuscitated" neurons gradually reconnect to the rest of the brain. These revived neurons and their connections help return the use of lost cerebral and bodily functions.

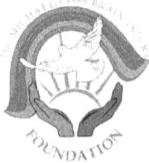

Hyperbaric therapy does not resurrect dead brain tissue, but it can facilitate the functioning of those dormant, idling nerve cells that have suffered secondary damage by stroke due to the diminished oxygen. Oftentimes, the brain area suffering secondary damage is a larger part of the brain, which suffered the primary damage. This area of secondary damage to the brain (the ischemic penumbra) is the area that HBOT helps.

Our Goals

1. To make brain injury survivors, as well as the family members, aware of the benefits of HBOT.
2. To organize fundraising activities to raise money to support the cost of HBOT.

3. With such therapy, to improve the quality of life of survivors of brain injuries and their family members.

Unfortunately, in our today's society governed by the power of money, not a chance is given to those who simply don't have the financial means to cover the cost of Hyperbaric Oxygenation Therapy treatments.

For example, a session can range from $100 to $150. Even though big improvements have been noticed in many survivors after ten to twenty sessions—even after months or years after the initial accident occurred—each survivor is a unique case and noticeable improvement can be different from one individual to another. An average of forty sessions is considered to be the minimum. Do the math and you will see that HBOT doesn't come cheap (a minimum of $4000 for forty treatments).

And HBOT for brain injury, just for many other medical conditions, is not covered by any insurance.

That's why our mission, until HBOT is approved for all these conditions (especially for TBI and ABI, and even beyond) will be to bring hope and financial help to those who cannot afford these treatments out of their own pockets.

The goal of this book isn't to raise money, but to instill hope in others and to raise awareness. I encourage you to visit my foundation website to learn more about TBI, about HBOT, and how you can make a difference. Please take a moment to visit SecondChanceStepbyStep.org to learn more.

Our First Honoree

September 7th, 2010, I had the real pleasure of meeting the first individual selected by our board of directors, who are all volunteers. They selected a young twelve –year-old girl by the name of Riley Skougard.

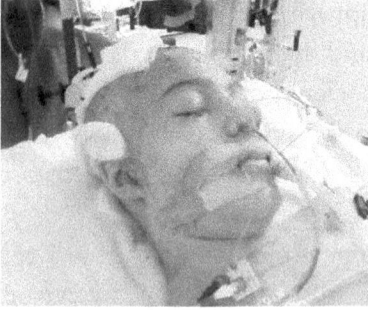

In November 2009, she began suffering from headaches, double vision, dizziness and nausea for about a week. She's twelve after all, and just got new prescription glasses, so there was no real cause for concern.

Then one evening, she suddenly lost consciousness. Rushed to the hospital, she was admitted to undergo an emergency brain surgery, during which she went into cardiac arrest for approximately thirty minutes before finally being revived. The doctors said she wouldn't make it through the night.

The doctors' best diagnosis was that a very rare condition called Arteriovenous Malformation (AVM) may have caused a rupture in her brain (similar to an aneurysm). But they aren't sure. More simply, she had bleeding in her brain. Since then, she has endured a series of brain surgeries (five in total) and has been in a coma since she first lost consciousness.

The Michael Coss Foundation will be assisting Riley with the initial eighty treatments of Hyperbaric Oxygen Therapy, at a value of $10,000. Without a doubt, these treatments will assist Riley in her recovery. The treating doctor, Dr. Zayd Ratansi, from the Advanced Hyperbaric Recovery Centre in Coquitlam, BC, is very positive and optimistic that her quality of life will be greatly improved from these treatments.

~Personal Essay~

Hi. My name is Sylvia Hoeree.

I met Mike in September of 2009 at his first fundraiser for the Michael Coss Foundation. What an honor to be part of this man's incredible journey. There are many words to describe this amazing man, but the one word that stands out to me is "determination."

The day I met Mike, I watched him slowly walk up to the podium with the assistance of a family member, and then I listened to him speak in front of a large crowd of people. His speech had been affected by his injury, but he touched everyone in the room that day.

He shared his tragic story with an added touch of humor and then shared his dreams to help other survivors. There was not one person in that room that believed he would fail.

"Without a doubt Mike will succeed."

I am proud to say that I am now friends with Mike, and volunteer for his foundation because I believe in him.

I have truly been blessed; I will be a witness to Mike's journey.

CHAPTER TEN

A Collection of Essays

*"The greatest healing therapy is
friendship and love."
-Hubert H. Humphrey, Jr.*

I felt it was important to include stories written from my closest friends, family members, and the caregivers I've had the pleasure to work with throughout my recovery. In many ways, their stories are much more profound than mine.

Each person has changed my life dramatically. They're a testament to my recovery and I'm so very grateful to be able to include their stories in this book and to have them in my life.

*****

My name is Joe Lozinski.

I met Mike Coss (Cosco) in 2000 at a Slow-pitch tournament in Langley. My wife Vanessa and I went out to play for John Stone, and we did not know anybody on the team. As it turned out, Mike and his brother Dwayne, over breakfast at the Golden Arches, had enticed Vanessa and me to come out and play more often.

They were truly a great and fun bunch of players, so eventually we went on a few road trips with the same people. This is a good story of how friendships are built. Kelowna, Penticton, Abbotsford and Whistler were some of the more common trips that became part of our summer tour.

After a few road trips together, Mike encouraged me to start our own ball team. Go figure, our team was called "Bad News Beers." To this day, Mike and I still discuss some of the road trips that we had been on. We've always had a special group of people on our team, and we never had any problem filling our roster when we required players. It did not matter if we won or lost, although it's always better to be on the winning side, our team would usually enjoy a tall cool one after the game. Mike had orchestrated many of these good times and good memories.

I remember the time when our team was playing in Abbotsford, and Mike had arranged to take a power boat and go tubing at Cultus Lake. This was in between games, and it is a boating trip I will never forget. This is one of the many stories of how Mike would go out of his way for the baseball team, hockey team, or workmates.

It's tough to find one word that describes Mike. Mike is always fun to be around. He is very positive and cheerful. He is fierce competitor in his own way, but most of all Mike is very "courageous."

Joe Lozinski, Coach

*****

Have you ever walked into a room of many people that you didn't know, and you find that you are drawn to one particular person?

Maybe he is smiling, laughing, or maybe it's just his charisma? He seems to be the life of the party, the one that everyone wants to get to know.

Well that's how I would describe Mike.

Hi, my name is Trish Martini, and I met Mike about twelve years ago while playing softball. Over the years we have played on the same softball team as well as the same ball hockey team. Mike is a great softball player, and with him on the team, it was always fun. He's an even better goalie—I would say he's the best goalie in the league, by far.

The one word I would use to describe Mike is "life." He is full of life, and he is always the life of the party. I am privileged to be his friend.

*****

Mike Coss—The Original

My first day in the beer business, I met Mike Coss. I was twenty two years old, fresh out of school and was a Field Marketing Assistant for Coors Light. My job that day was to work the computer for a presentation that several of the Molson reps were doing for a customer.

Mike Coss was one of the presenters. I remember looking up at him thinking, 'man, this guy can talk.'

The customer was clearly impressed with Mike, and I think it helped that he said her name every twenty seconds or so, 'So, you see Sue, if you were to reassemble for cooler doors, here are the potential profit outcomes, Sue.'

I was impressed too. He was very convincing and likable from a first meeting.

I worked with Cosco that summer and the summer after. I worked with him more than anyone else as he always presented a case as to why he needed more help than the other reps. That was fine with me because Cosco always treated me like a friend.

Don't get me wrong, he wasn't shy to ask me to work, and work hard. He even asked me bring him a 'Double Double and an Old Fashion Plain' every morning. I cleaned out his notorious lockers, filled sky high with Molson wearable's and swag. I well understood his nickname 'Cosco'.

It wasn't the most glamorous of jobs, but I was always rewarded for my efforts. Cosco always showed everyone, including me, his appreciation. I watched in awe as he turned some of the most sceptical of customers into believers. Of course, the doughnuts helped and so did Cosco's charm.

From a professional standpoint, Cosco is one of the best salespeople the beer business has ever seen. He holds closely the human qualities that draw people to him, to trust him and ultimately make them want to buy whatever he is selling. I looked up to him for this and still work to emulate some of these qualities that came so naturally to Cosco.

As much as I admired Cosco for being such a great salesperson, I really admired his incredible love of family. Cosco is a family person. He would talk about Annie all the time and would share with me his dreams to have a family. I remember the day he told me that Annie was pregnant, with twins! He was thrilled. And as we sat there and watched the game together I looked at Cosco and saw a whole new happiness that radiated from within. In all his happiness, however, he still worried about his dog Murph being jealous, as Murph was treated as good as a family member would be.

When Cosco got hurt, I, along with everyone else who knew him, was devastated. Admittedly, I had to muster up the courage to go and see him at the hospital. It was very difficult and unfortunately I was only able to do it once. While there, I watched Annie and saw her smile and put on a brave face. She would talk to Cosco, touch him, and do anything in her power to create a reaction. I have never seen a woman fight so hard and be as strong as Annie. She is amazing.

Now that Cosco is on the long and difficult road to recovery, I see a relentless determination from within. He has resolved to achieve his goal of walking again. I believe that if anyone can do it, it's Cosco. I know that Cosco will keep up his driven spirit and will find success in all he does. He is a winner, a fighter, and most importantly, a wonderful human being.

*****

Michael was in a motor vehicle accident in the summer of 2006. Without warning and without his permission, Michael's life changed forever. He sustained a brain injury and has for the past two and a half years been involved in extensive physical and cognitive rehabilitation. He has demonstrated a remarkable recovery and has overcome many challenges.

No two brains are alike, and therefore no two injured brains are alike. Brain injury is not black and white. There is not an easy fix program. Adjusting to change requires the confidence to let go of what was and the courage to explore what is still to come.

None of us are exempt from experiencing a sudden life change, regardless of whether change is forced on us or whether we choose it. Jobs end, companies re-organize, children grow up and leave home, and accidents happen. In Michael's situation, he experienced a sudden life change after his motor vehicle accident.

Michael knows firsthand about the painful process of accepting change. Michael is learning practical strategies to help him let go of his fears, eliminate his resistance, and to change and move forward in a positive direction. Michael is learning step by step strategies to gain the physical strength to walk again.

Michael arrived in one of our community-based group homes in February 2007.

He was just emerging from a coma. He was unaware of his surroundings. He required total care support and had extensive contractures of all his limbs. He was not expected to recover beyond his present condition, to be independent, or to walk again. Michael went through various stages of recovery from awakening to the vital person he is today.

His rehabilitation program has been comprehensive, providing a wide array of services from a multidisciplinary team which includes physical therapy. The physical therapy program has been designed to identify problem areas and to develop strategies for Michael that would produce positive results, such as a new way to walk or to be mobile.

Michael is a fighter. He has worked diligently on his physical rehabilitation every day which has included strengthening, stretching, balance and gait training, bed mobility, transfer training, and coordination. As a result, he is regaining physical strength and endurance and is, much to the surprise of most professionals, walking today.

The process has been slow, but progress steady and he is deserving of recognition for the demanding and tedious work he has done to get where he is today. He has accomplished his goal of walking again, and just needs to continue to practice his new skill to make walking more habitual.

Physical rehabilitation is hard work and the rewards are slow and difficult to see. However, Michael is making the most out of life after his brain injury. He gets up every day in a positive frame of mind and dedicates his day to his rehabilitation. He does whatever it takes to hold on and to regain back his physical ability. He keeps positive and motivated and believing that tomorrow will be better. Michael uses a wheelchair, which serves as a reminder that the injury occurred. He is not accepting the fact that he will not walk again and is working hard every day on his physical therapy rehabilitation.

Michael is living testimony to how a successful man can be knocked down but not out, and how to overcome and succeed no matter what life throws his way. Michael is working on accepting the new person he has become, with a whole new outlook on life and knowing that he is a vital member of his community with much to offer. I am so impressed by his courage, his attitude, his perseverance, and his positive outlook for each challenge he faces every day.

I have been touched by his determination and motivation, his playful spirit, and his positive outlook on life. Michael's personal experience translates into lessons we can all learn from. Never lose hope, never give up, stay positive, and make positive change for yourself.

I believe that Michael embodies the following message: change the changeable, accept the unchangeable and remove yourself from the unacceptable. One day Michael wants to be a motivational speaker to share his experiences with others and to help other survivors. I believe he will accomplish this, and in doing so will definitely be giving back to his community.

From the first time you meet Michael, your life will be transformed in a positive way. His life is intertwined with hope, courage, and is an inspiration to other survivors. Mike has overcome some major obstacles since his car accident and has made a choice to make the best of some really tough situations.

He does and will continue to make an impact on people's lives with his continued story.

Sue McCrimmon
Cheshire Homes Society of B.C. (2009)

*****

Hi Mike, I cannot recall too much about the time you worked at the clinic, but I sure remember the time you took off on my old Triumph! I had gone to show you my then new, now old, bike, when you asked me if you could take it for a ride. I knew that you could ride a motorcycle, but the difference with the Triumph is that the rear brake and the gear shifter are on the opposite side compared to the motorcycles of today. I have to admit that I was a little reluctant at first because I was afraid that you would end up dans le decor.

So after explaining how to first of all start the bike, because there is no starter on a 1968 Triumph Tiger 100(500cc), you have to kick start it, not only did the bike start, but it started on the first kick. It usually took me two to four kicks to get the motor to start.

After giving you the usual precautions, off you went. Honestly I was expecting to hear the gears screech because you have to really pull in the clutch and time your gear change in order that everything changes smoothly. Well, to my surprise that's exactly what happened! I guess you had inherited your father's genes! When you came back, you had a big smile on your face, and so did I.

To my surprise, you had ridden that bike like you had always been able to. So, big boy, that's the time you had impressed me the most.

Of course, I never saw how you" cruised" the women. You probably would have impressed me even more!

Have a nice day, love you big boy, Norman.

*****

My name is Linda Thomas.

I worked at Molson (based out of Calgary) at the same time as Mike, leading the Customer Marketing team of which Mike was a key member. We didn't work together for very long before Mike's accident, but I had the good fortune to have dinner with Mike and a few others at a Sales Conference in Montreal a few months prior.

That was where I really got to know Mike, and I left that dinner impressed with him as an employee, but also as a person. Mike's energy filled the table and engaged us all. His passion for his work was evident to everyone.

We talked about his move to Vancouver, and the loves of his life—Annie and the kids. He shared pictures. He talked about his aspirations both at work and in his personal life. I left that evening quite certain that I, and many others, would all be working for Mike one day—he had leadership qualities that would take him far in life.

And we see those now, although not in the way that I envisioned that evening in Montreal. Through Mike's life experiences since that time, he has demonstrated personal strength and leadership in ways well beyond what I ever envisioned. He has touched the lives of so many people, including me.

I can't begin to express my respect and admiration for his personal strength, perseverance, and positive outlook. Mike has inspired countless people, many that he doesn't even know, to be better.

If there were people like Mike in the world, it would be a better place. I am honoured and privileged to have known him.

Sincerely,
Linda Thomas

*****

My name is Jeff Armstrong.

I have had the pleasure to know Mike since he started with Molson, which was many moons ago! I was in the process of moving from BC to Toronto when we hired Cosco, so my day-to-day interactions were few, but the occasions we shared were not only enjoyable but also impressionable.

I recall vividly the first of my In Market Coaching days with Cosco. The purpose of the day was to identify best practices of our Sales Professionals and, if required, identify areas of opportunity for development. It was not only one of the most enjoyable days I've had with a rep, but I also left with two lasting impressions.

First, the day was delayed as, if I recall correctly, something had happened to his cell phone preventing him from being accessible. He was quick to make alternative plans. Shortly into the day, Mike revealed that he and his wife Ann were in the process of creating babies, and in the midst of some emotional times. He was distracted, to say the least, as being out of contact on this day was not part of the plan. Right then, I knew this was a special person. He could have easily cancelled the day, but I discovered a lasting insight to his character that day: Here was a man extremely committed to his family, focused on his job, and someone who would go to great lengths to balance the two.

As the day went on, it became abundantly clear I was only collecting best practices for other Sales Champions to aspire to. In particular, Mike is textbook when it comes to summarizing and understanding customer needs, but his ability to wrap up a sales call by confirming quantities, identifying next steps, and detailing timing was second to none.

Not stopping there though, Mike consistently used his flawless wrap-up to always ASK for something else. That one little additional thing that on its own wouldn't amount to much, but when accumulated makes the difference between good and great.

I could use many words to describe Cosco…passionate, focused, committed, consistent, and professional, but I choose to best describe Mike as "memorable." Mike is memorable in his ability to fight for the quality of life he desires for his family and is memorable in his professional selling abilities that, to this day, I incorporate his 'flawless wrap-up' to my training sessions with future Sales Champions.

Jeff 'Army' Armstrong
Director—Sales Training, Molson Coors Canada

*****

Hi there, my name is Jennifer McCreath.

Mike and I met about nine years ago while I was working at Sammy J. Peppers. I was in charge of promotions and special events there, so I met Mike through some of the programs we did with Molson.

When I left Sammy's to start my own promotions company, Platinum Ambition, Mike was a very supportive friend and gave Tash and me a lot of direction in the industry. He provided us with a lot of business contacts by bringing us along on golf outings and to promotional events.

From judging bikini contests to sampling Molson products in pubs, he definitely gave us a serious leg up in the growth of our business. My favourite event would have to be the golf and sturgeon fishing tournament at the Sand Piper golf course. It was a fabulous day spent with good friends and cold beer.

I unwittingly made the day much more exciting when I fell off the back of the jet boat into the Fraser River, which forced about four or five fishing boats to race to my rescue after pulling their lines. I believe our team was awarded for catching the most unusual fish.

If I had one word to describe Mike, it would be "charismatic." His energy, passion and focus are something I truly admire and respect. His dedication to his family and his work has always been something to look up to, and I am proud to say that I've learned a lot from him.

Mike's smile and never ending energy have always been such a breath of fresh air and he is someone that I am proud to say is and always will be a very dear friend!

Jen McCreath

*****

Je m'appelle Karine Fortin et j'ai connue Mike il y a environ 10 ans alors que nous travaillons ensemble pour RBH Inc. La compagnie a perdu un très gros joueur lorsqu'il a décidé de réorienter sa carrière et de partir chez Molson Coors Canada. Même si on ne se voit pas souvent, nous avons toujours gardé contact, Mike est une personne sur qui je sais que je peux compter car une fois que tu fais parti de ses amis (es) tu es dans sa vie pour toujours.

Il était là pour nous lorsque nous avons été travailler à Vancouver, il nous a permis de vivre l'expérience du Grand Prix avec tout le glamour que cela englobe et j'étais très contente d'avoir la chance de le revoir même si nous ne sommes plus collègues. Sa famille compte énormément pour lui, rien n'est plus important à ses yeux et je suis fière de tout ce qu'il a accompli avant et après son accident.

Si je devais décrire Mike en un seul mot (je suis une femme, c'est quand même un peu difficile!!!) je dirais "persévérant."

Il se donne à fond dans tout ce qu'il entreprend, il ne lâche jamais et atteint toujours les buts qu'il se fixe autant dans sa vie personnelle que professionnelle.

Chapeau Mike, je suis très heureuse de te connaître!!!

English Translation:
My name is Karine Fortin, I met Mike about ten years ago when we were both working for RBH inc. The company lost a very good employee when he decided to work for Molson. We always stayed in touch. Mike is a person that you can count on. When you are his friend, it is forever.

Nothing is more important for him than his family, and I am very proud of everything he has accomplished before and after his accident.

One word to describe Mike would be PERSEVERANCE.

When he undertakes something, he gives a hundred percent of himself. He never gives up and always succeeds in obtaining his objectives (personal and professional).

I am very happy to know you and I raise my hat to you.

*****

My name is Denis Richer.

I am a Business Development Representative for Rothmans Benson & Hedges. I have been with this company for the last seventeen years. I want to tell you about my friend Mike Coss. The first time I met Mike, we were both attending the first National Personal Best Award for the RBH Company.

I work in the province of Québec and Mike was working in British Columbia. The first thing that struck me is that I was faced with a guy working in BC that was very fluent in French. It did not take too long to find out that this was not his only asset. I discovered a man with a desire to win, to do a good job, and that had been brought up with solid values.

The year after, in our second annual meeting, he was named the rep of the year for the province of British Columbia. I don't have to tell you that I was not surprised. Mike left the company a few years later to join the Molson Breweries. I thought I was done with the Coss family, but no, Mike's brother, Dwayne was also named as rep of the year for the province of BC.

A couple of years later, in jest, I said to Mike that Mike had been cloned. Mike and I kept in touch, and I had the opportunity to work in BC for a couple of weeks to launch a new product. As soon as I found out, I called Mike and we made arrangements to meet while I was in Vancouver.

It just so happened that the Molson Indy was being held in Vancouver on the weekend I was staying over. Mike being with Molson's, I asked him if he had any tickets for the race. He treated me with a couple of VIP passes for the race, which turned out to be one of the best weekends I had ever spent.

Then came the bad news. I was devastated when I heard about the accident and the extent of the injuries to Mike, but was glad to see that his family was OK. But you know what, I knew that he would one day recover and that he would overcome all the challenges of a recovery.

As I write this today, I have just heard that Mike walked in the hallway the other day. What a giant step! Mike and I do not get to see each other often, but we stay in contact via email. Even though we are far apart, I think about Mike just about every day and I can tell you that when things are getting tough, he is my inspiration.

*****

My name is Doug Rutz and my son's name is Travis.

Travis was severally injured in a race car accident in Sept 2009 at a dirt track in Indiana. Since then, I have met a lot of other family's with similar cases. One of the truly bright spots in what has been a very depressing time for us was meeting Michael.

We met Michael and his family at Coquitlam Hyperbaric while taking oxygen treatments. Every once in a while, Michael would show up for a visit and when he did, he would light up the room. His passion for life and energy has inspired us so much to keep going forward.

To say that Michael was the highlight of the day would be an understatement. My son is now about eight months out from his accident and is moving forward every day, and like Michael says, we are training for a marathon. Some good things can come about in these tragic situations, and Michael has been one of those. I am honoured and proud to call him my friend.

Doug Rutz

*****

Resources

The Michael Coss Brain Injury Foundation:
www.secondchancestepbystep.com
You can also find me on Facebook:
The Courage to Come Back (Michael Coss)

For more information about Traumatic Brain Injury:
traumaticbraininjury.com

Historical Archives; Find out what happened on any day, anywhere, any time: historyorb.com

For more information about HBOT visit the fine folks at www.hyperbaricexperts.com. You can grab their free brain report at http://www.hyperbaricexperts.com/report/Free%20Brain%20Report-July%2024-09-FINAL.pdf

And for more information on the Stand Up For Mental Health program visit: http://www.standupformentalhealth.com/about.shtml

Finally, for more information about CONNECT Communities, homes, and support after brain injury, visit: www.connectcommunities.ca

www.ingramcontent.com/pod-product-compliance
Lightning Source LLC
Chambersburg PA
CBHW072255270326
41930CB00010B/2383